The
American
Cancer
Society

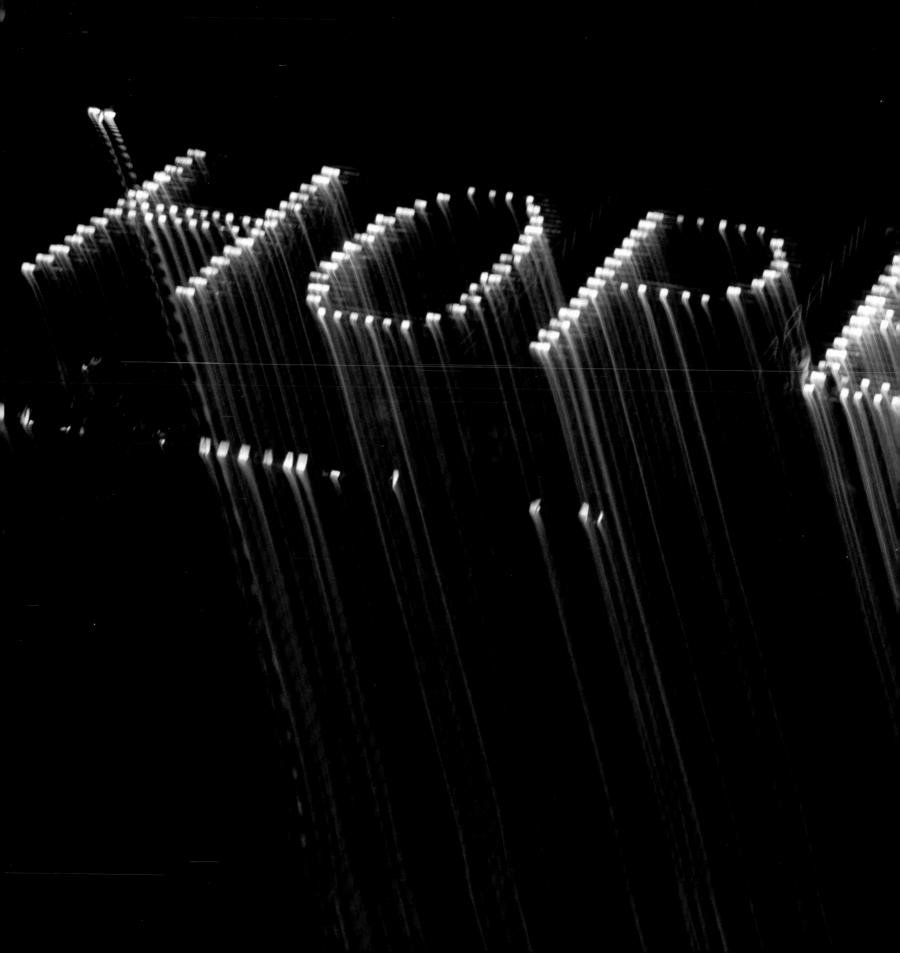

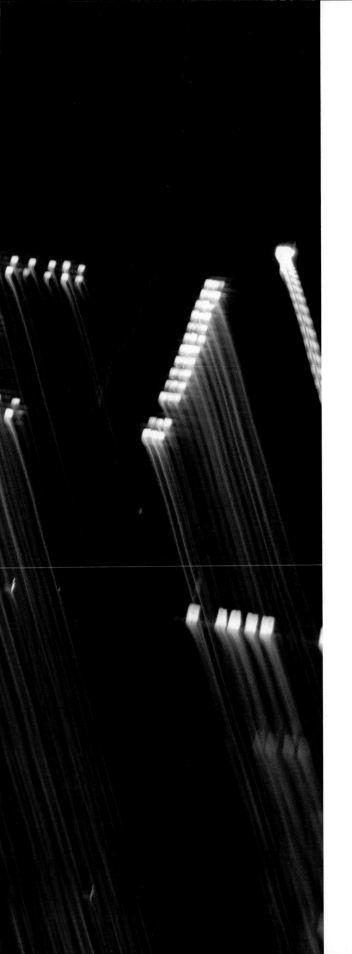

The

American Cancer Society

A History of Saving Lives

Foreword by George H. W. Bush

Written by Irvin Fleming, MD,
and Harmon Eyre, MD,
with Jan Pogue

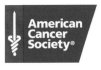

Published by the
American Cancer Society
250 Williams Street NW
Atlanta, Georgia 30303
800-227-2345
cancer.org

Strategic Director, Content: Chuck Westbrook
Director, Book Publishing: Len Boswell
Managing Editor, Books: Rebecca Teaff, MA
Marketing/Rights Manager, Books: Candace Magee
Publishing Coordinator, Books: Vanika Jordan, MSPub
Editor, Books: Jill Russell
Editorial Assistant, Books: Amy Rovere

BOOKHOUSE
GROUP, INC.

Book Development by
Bookhouse Group, Inc.
818 Marietta Street NW
Atlanta, Georgia 30318
404-885-9515
www.bookhouse.net

Editorial Director: Rob Levin
Managing Editor: Sarah Edwards Fedota
Chief Operating Officer: Renee Peyton
Book and Cover Design: Laurie Shock
Copy Editing and Indexing: Bob Land
Prepress: Jill Dible

10 11 12 13 14   5 4 3 2 1

Manufactured in Canada

Library of Congress Cataloging-in-Publication Data

Fleming, Irvin D.
  The American Cancer Society : a history of saving lives / written by Irvin
Fleming and Harmon Eyre with Jan Pogue.
     p. cm.
  "Foreword by George H. W. Bush."
  ISBN-13: 978-0-944235-91-1 (alk. paper)
  ISBN-10: 0-944235-91-3 (alk. paper)
  1. American Cancer Society—History. 2. Cancer—United States—History.
I. Eyre, Harmon J. II. Pogue, Jan. III. Title.

  RC276. F64 2009
  362.196′99400973—dc22
                              2008023593

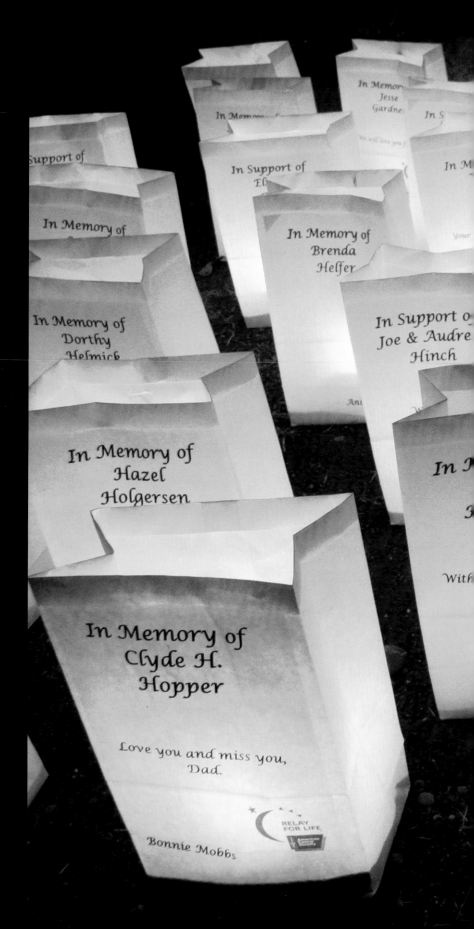

Right: Luminaria at an American Cancer Society Relay For Life® event

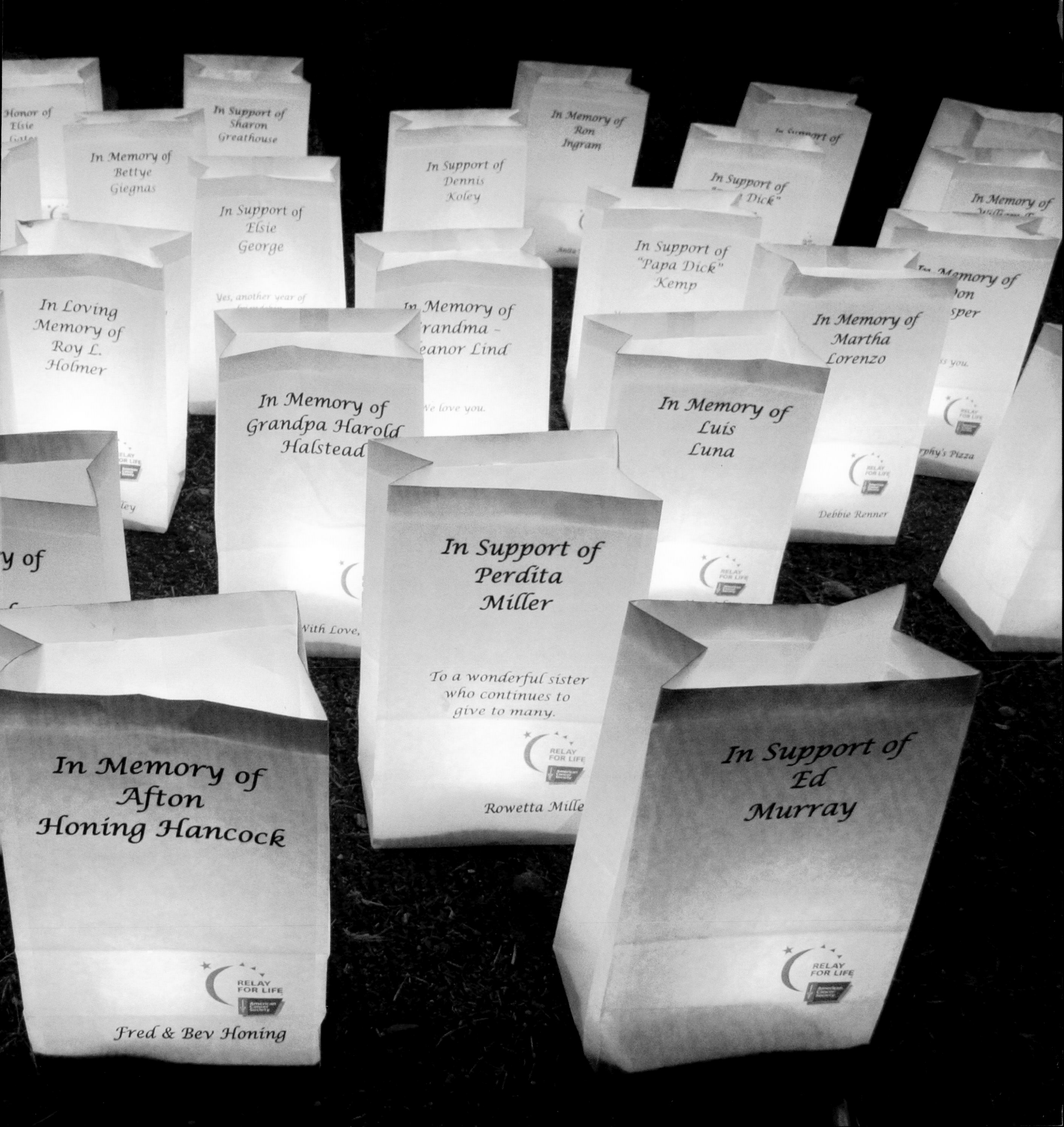
In Support of
Sharon
Greathouse
In Memory of
Bettye
Giegnas
In Support of
Dennis
Koley
In Memory of
Ron
Ingram
In Support of
Elsie
George
In Support of
"Papa Dick"
Kemp
In Loving
Memory of
Roy L.
Holmer
In Memory of
Martha
Lorenzo
In Memory of
Grandpa Harold
Halstead
We love you.
In Memory of
Luis
Luna
Debbie Renner
In Support of
Perdita
Miller
To a wonderful sister
who continues to
give to many.
RELAY
FOR LIFE
In Memory of
Afton
Honing Hancock
In Support of
Ed
Murray
RELAY
FOR LIFE
Fred & Bev Honing
RELAY
FOR LIFE

Acknowledgments

The time and efforts of many people made this project possible. Special thanks to Dr. John Seffrin for his review and valuable input.

For assistance with research and images, thanks to Sarah Assalti, Craig Combs, Meggan Hood, Nicol Jimerson, Brooke Kennett, Jean Nichols, Margaret Rogers, Kristen Sullivan, Dana Wagner, Betsy Wallace, and Sondra Wright.

We are grateful to Sarah Fedota and the staff of Bookhouse Group for shepherding the book through to completion.

In addition to those listed here, many others gave valuable information and shared their experiences and memories. We appreciate the efforts and assistance of all who helped to create this book and all of those whose work has been in support of the mission of the American Cancer Society: to eliminate cancer as a major health problem by preventing cancer, saving lives, and diminishing suffering from cancer, through research, education, advocacy, and service.

SUPERVISING EDITOR
Jill Russell

PERMISSIONS EDITOR
Vanika Jordan, MSPub

ART ADVISOR
Tom Deal

CONTRIBUTING RESEARCHER
Jeff Clements

EDITOR
Emily Pualwan

CONTRIBUTING EDITORS
Michelle Boone
Crystal Garrick

EDITORIAL ASSISTANT
Amy Rovere

REVIEWERS

Sherry Bailey
Dileep G. Bal
Linelle Blais
Michelle Boone
Otis Brawley
Helene Brown
Jeff Clements
Marty Coelho
Francis Coolidge
Tom Deal
Greg Donaldson
Allan Erickson
Pat Felts
Patricia Flynn
Crystal Garrick
Tom Glynn
Sheffield Hale
Mike Heron
Kay Horsch

Harry Johns
John Laszlo
Ray Lenhard
Len Lichtenfeld
LaMar McGinnis
Marion Morra
Terry Music
Emily Pualwan
Irv Reimer
David Rosenthal
Steve Sener
Mary Simmonds
Dan Smith
John Stevens
Gary Streit
Don Thomas
Michael Thun
Gerald Woolam

Contents

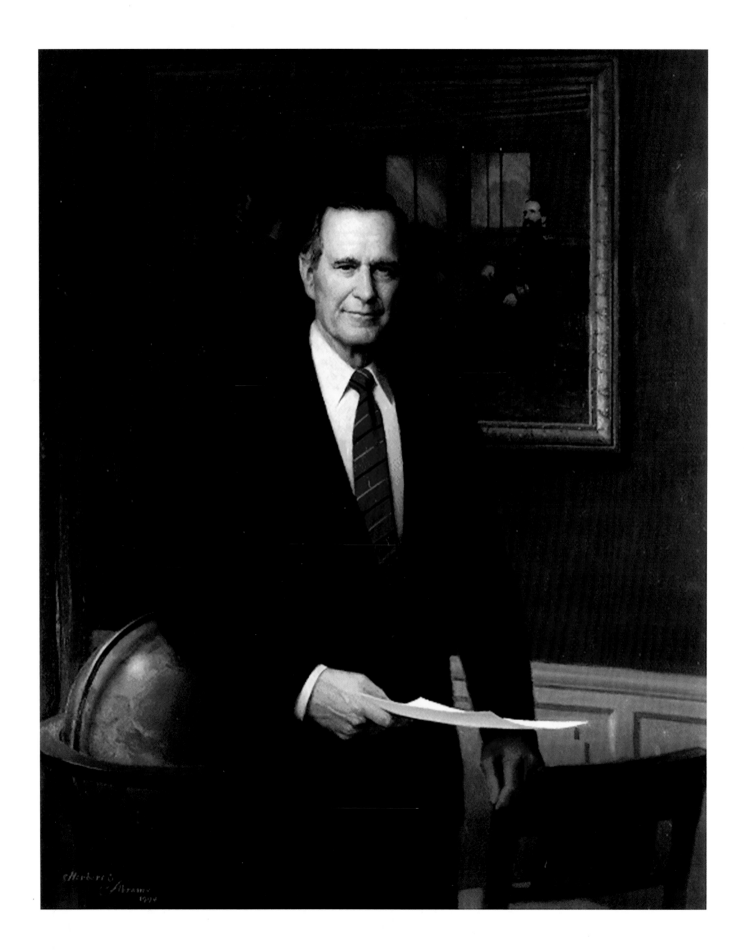

Foreword

By President George H. W. Bush

The American Society for the Control of Cancer was founded in 1913 by a small group of physicians and businessmen and one woman who recognized the importance of providing accurate and timely information about cancer to both the medical community and the public. Their first meeting, which took place at the Harvard Club in New York City, was described by one founding member as "the inauguration of a moment . . . that will be of the greatest importance in the investigation of cancer."

Those words were prophetic, and their mission is still being carried out, fostering a greater legacy than the founding members could have imagined. Known today as the American Cancer Society, the organization counts among its achievements the sponsorship of forty-four investigators who went on to receive the Nobel Prize. And the Society remains true to its original purpose. At its core, it remains a grassroots, community-based coalition of volunteers committed to eliminating cancer as a major health threat worldwide.

A Personal Note

The fight against cancer has been a major focus of my personal and professional life. In 1953, my wife, Barbara, and I lost our four-year-old daughter, Robin, to leukemia. In those days, survival rates were very low, and despite various medical treatments, our beloved daughter died. Afterward, we vowed to use any opportunities available to us to improve the lives of people touched by cancer, to find ways to combat the disease, and to spare other families the grief we had experienced. We made a commitment to honor our daughter by raising awareness of the disease so that other children would have a chance to live. Today, with early detection methods and improved medical treatments, many children and adults diagnosed with cancer will have a good chance of surviving and living a full, active life.

Opposite: Official White House portrait of President George H. W. Bush

Fighting Cancer with Knowledge

In some ways, our family's experience and that of so many others in our situation mirrors the struggle of the American Cancer Society throughout its own history—to fight cancer with knowledge. When the Society was founded almost a century ago, there was not only a paucity of information available about the disease, but much of what was believed was false. In 1905, a survey by the American Medical Association found that most Americans, even some physicians, believed that a diagnosis of cancer was a death sentence and any action was useless. The word "cancer" held a stigma so powerful that families hid the disease and begged their doctors to keep the diagnosis off death certificates. Even by 1919, when President Warren G. Harding wrote an endorsement letter for "National Cancer Week," he did not mention the word "cancer" but called it "this particular disease." Thus, in its early days, the American Cancer Society bore the weight of a tremendous burden. To overcome that burden, it adopted a simple mission: to gather facts and educate the public.

One Person Can Make a Difference

Early in its history, the Society determined that its executive committee should include men and women from an equal number of lay and medical/scientific professions. The president of the organization would always be a scientist or physician, and the chair of the board would always be a layperson. Diversity in its leadership has certainly contributed to the Society's success, but it has also depended on the talents, dedication, and sheer will of many individuals. As I read this history, I was struck by the fact that many of the amazing achievements in cancer research and treatment were made possible because one individual—often at a crucial juncture—stepped up and made a difference.

Among those individuals are many dynamic women who advanced the cause. For example, Mary Lasker, the wife of a prominent advertising executive, staged a successful fundraising campaign for cancer research in the 1940s, even while America was at war. Before Mary Lasker's campaign, the Society had not allocated one penny to cancer research, but by 1947, donations exceeded twelve million dollars. There were other women like Helene Brown, who learned in 1950 that a Pap test could save women's lives; she would subsequently spend more than fifty years as a leading public health advocate and Society volunteer.

There were physicians such as J. Marion Sims, who was fired from the staff of the Woman's Hospital of New York in 1874 after refusing to deny hospital admission to cancer patients. There were scientists such as Clarence Cook Little, who officially formed the Women's Field Army in 1937, the group that would distribute two million pieces of literature to educate the public about cancer in 1943 alone and that would raise almost all the money supporting the Society for nearly a decade.

A New Medical Specialty

Not until the 1950s did oncology come to the forefront as a new medical specialty. The American Cancer Society recognized that progress in research would depend on a critical mass of physician-investigators who were studying cancer and its causes and developing better treatments. Thus, the Society began to provide funding for young researchers at a time when little funding was available from other sources. Those research dollars have led to phenomenal discoveries by luminaries such as Sidney Farber, whose work started the era of chemotherapy; Charles Huggins, whose Nobel Prize–winning research changed forever the way scientists regarded the behavior of all cancer cells; and James Watson, who, with research partner Francis Crick, discovered DNA's double-helix structure.

In addition to funding research, the Society recognized that studies of specific groups were needed to understand and fight the disease. Before the Society started its first epidemiology department in 1946, national mortality statistics had shown an alarming 500 percent increase in lung cancer deaths over a sixteen-year period. Society-sponsored epidemiologic studies would lead to important findings, such as confirming the link between tobacco smoking and lung cancer. Though such a link seems obvious today, it had to be proved by rigorous scientific study.

When the Society launched its first Cancer Prevention Study in 1959, it supplied key data for the reports on smoking and health issued by the surgeon general's office. Succeeding projects would reveal an astonishing increase in lung cancer among women and add to our knowledge of how various medications, medical conditions, familial factors, and environmental exposures may affect cancer risk. By the 1990s, the Society's leadership had begun to appreciate and study the inherent, environmental, and cultural factors that have an impact on human behavior, particularly in people's perceptions, and how they could be influenced through education. These data have provided the base for many of the Society's campaigns—from anti-smoking to the right for more universal access to health care.

A Global Reach

Over the years, the influence of the American Cancer Society has been far reaching—not only in America but throughout the world. Barbara and I witnessed this firsthand in the summer of 2006 when we attended the World Cancer Congress in Washington, D.C. The meeting was sponsored by the American Cancer Society and the International Union Against Cancer (UICC). We were there as cochairs of C-Change, a consortium of leaders from business, government, and nonprofit organizations who share a vision of a future where cancer is prevented, detected early, and cured, or managed successfully as a chronic illness. The World Cancer Congress and a succeeding conference on tobacco control drew thousands of international cancer and tobacco control leaders from more than 130 countries.

The American Cancer Society has come a long way since the early days of the twentieth century when cancer—"this particular disease"—was so misunderstood. Scientists and physicians have now attained the knowledge to save lives, but the cancer burden is still one of epidemic proportion, especially in developing nations. In the United States, a milestone was achieved in 2006, with news of the first decline in the actual number of cancer deaths since national mortality record keeping was instituted in 1930. There is hope, but progress depends on a continuing global outreach.

Constituents of the American Cancer Society—cancer survivors and their loved ones; concerned citizens; advocacy groups; government, corporate, and community leaders; and health care specialists—will continue to support the mission and move the organization forward. If you are holding this book right now, there is a good chance you or someone you love has received a cancer diagnosis. In the lives of cancer patients, you know that every contribution—a hospital visit, a meal delivered, a dollar donated, a Relay walked—does make a difference. My hope is that, milestone by milestone, nation by nation, we will one day see the elimination of cancer as a major health problem for this and future generations.

This history was written not only to serve as an archive of the American Cancer Society's growth and achievements over the last ninety-six years, but to honor those individuals who have advanced knowledge in the field of cancer research and continue working every day toward easing the burden of cancer and finding a cure. Anyone who has been affected by cancer, as well as those who have devoted their lives to finding a cure for the disease, will find this a compelling and inspiring narrative.

— President George H. W. Bush

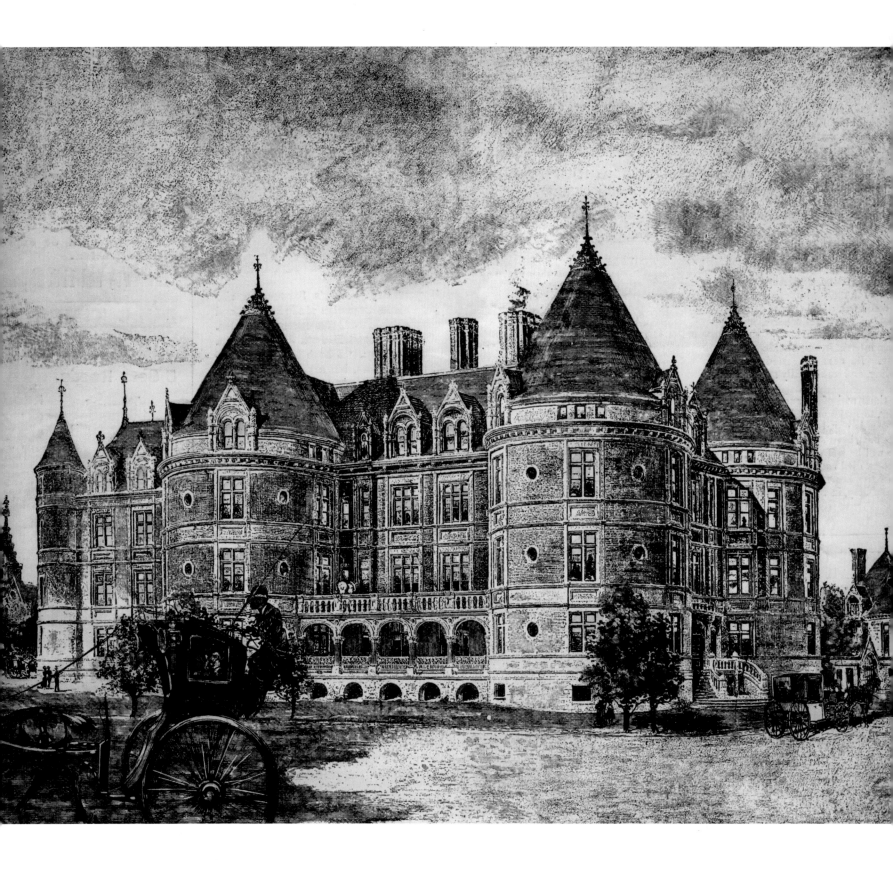

Introduction

Morphine and champagne. Carriage rides in Central Park. Sunday services in the hospital's Chapel of Saint Elizabeth of Hungary, named for the patron saint of the suffering.

For the patients admitted to the New York Cancer Hospital after it opened in 1887—so aptly named, so poorly received because of that name—treatment for their incurable diseases was an attempt to keep pain at bay, spirits high, and God near.

The hospital, funded by members of an elite New York City family itself ravaged by cancer, was an open attempt to fight the stigma of a disease so unmentionable that families hid their sick from neighbors and begged their doctors to keep the diagnosis off death certificates. Most hospitals would not accept cancer patients, and most physicians considered cancer patients incurable and possibly contagious; special care was often given to the dishes and linens of a cancer patient because of fear of contagion.

As historian David Cantor put it in 1993, "If cancer were both a product of and a danger to industrial and urban society . . . then individuals who had the diseases may themselves somehow be responsible for the social disorder."

New York Cancer Hospital, the first specialized cancer hospital in America, was a direct assault on these beliefs.

Charlotte Augusta Astor and her cousin, Elizabeth Cullum, were the forces behind the building of the New York Cancer Hospital. Both women were members of the influential Ladies' Board of the Woman's Hospital, a medical center begun in 1855 by thirty wealthy women who wanted a hospital exclusively for women. Dr. J. Marion Sims, a surgeon eventually credited as being the "father of gynecology," practiced there. Sims was particularly noted for a surgical cure for women with a painful and previously incurable disorder that sometimes followed childbirth. Yet he had from the beginning of his career been interested in the plight of cancer patients, particularly women with uterine cancer. Slowly, he began accepting cancer patients to the Woman's Hospital.

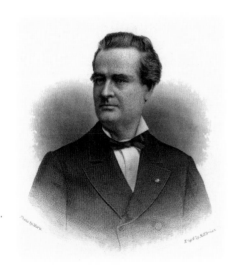

Elizabeth Cullum

Opposite: The New York Cancer Hospital opened its doors in 1887 and was the first facility of its kind in the United States to treat and care for cancer patients. Above: Dr. J. Marion Sims, the "father of gynecology," was a founder of the Woman's Hospital in New York. Above right: Elizabeth Cullum, granddaughter of Alexander Hamilton, was a force behind the founding of the New York Cancer Hospital. Her son died of cancer around the time the hospital opened its doors.

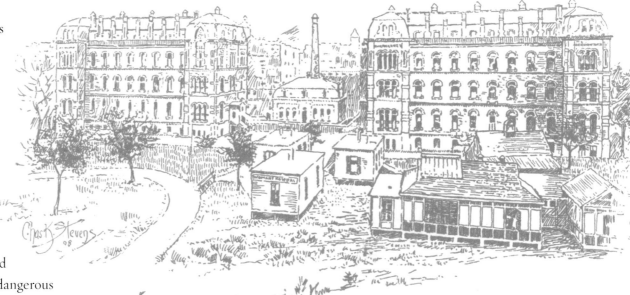

Admitting patients with such a scandalous disease went directly against the beliefs of the ladies of the board, who raised funds and oversaw the running of the hospital. The women, like many Americans in the mid-nineteenth century, believed cancer was not only dangerous and contagious but might be caused by venereal disease—and certainly was more appropriate for discussion in the boudoir than the drawing room. When Sims installed two patients with cancer in the open wards, the women leaders of the hospital detailed their complaints to him by noting he was "causing great discomfort and danger to the other patients in the ward." Eventually, the Ladies' Board ordered Sims to banish all cancer victims and hired a guard to stand at the entrance of the operating room to scrutinize his patients. In doing this, they cited "their mission of work and love as moral agents in the supervision of the hospital," and noted that, despite their best efforts, "a death occurred from cancer, which case caused extreme annoyance and suffering in all patients."

The battle was eventually both lost and won: Sims was summarily kicked out of the hospital in 1874 for refusing to deny cancer patients treatment. Two years after his exclusion from the hospital, Sims was elected president of the American Medical Association. In 1882, he was invited to again join the Woman's Hospital as a consulting surgeon—and was promptly expelled again when he insisted on treating cancer patients. He died, distinguished and admired by those in cancer research, in 1883.

Augusta Astor, an unusually progressive and broad-minded woman, watched the fight over treatment of cancer patients with interest. Her husband anonymously tendered an offer to the Woman's Hospital in 1883 for one hundred eighty thousand dollars to build a pavilion wing for the treatment of cancer patients. The offer was declined by the Ladies' Board, and the Astors dropped the offer.

Elizabeth Cullum, Augusta's beautiful and vivacious cousin, served with her on the

Above: The New York Woman's Hospital where, twice, Dr. J. Marion Sims was forced to leave his position as surgeon for refusing to turn away cancer patients. Below: Augusta Astor prodded her husband, John Jacob, to offer a substantial contribution to the Woman's Hospital in 1883, but the offer was declined. Eventually, her attention turned to the New York Cancer Hospital.

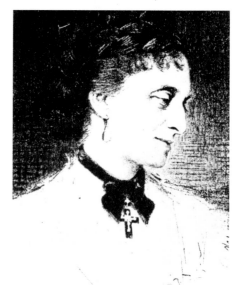

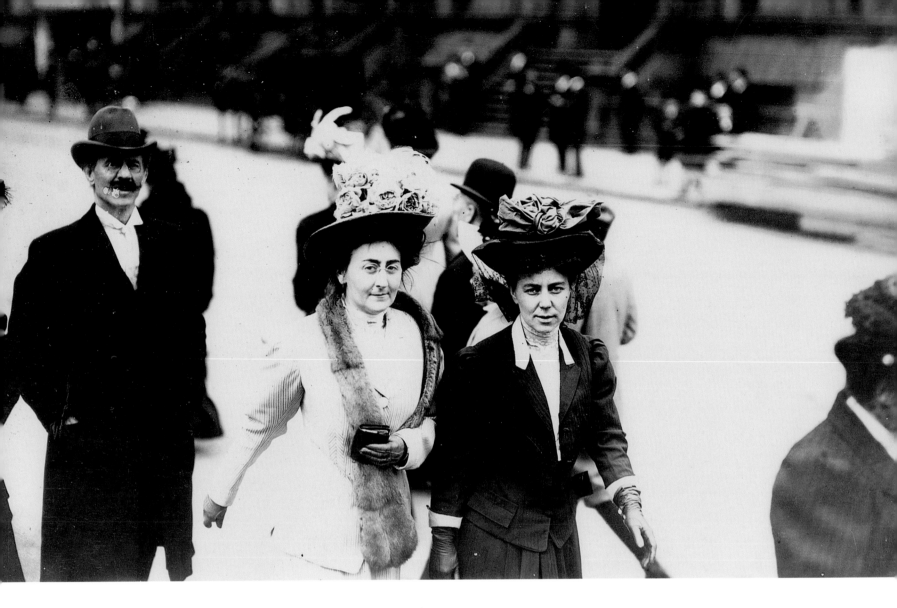

Above: In the late nineteenth century, many Americans regarded cancer as shameful and contagious. Most were afraid to be treated in the same facility as cancer patients.

hospital's Ladies' Board. She was the grand-daughter of Alexander Hamilton and the widow of the general-in-chief of the Union Army during the early days of the Civil War. Years after the war's end, she remarried another general, a man who had worked to improve the medical department of the Army of the Potomac and who became one of the nine charter members of the U.S. Sanitary Commission, forerunner of the American Red Cross.

In the spring of 1882, one year before Astor made the anonymous offer to fund a pavilion for the hospital, Mrs. Cullum's only child, Henry, died of cancer. As always, the word never appeared publicly. That fall, she herself began to show symptoms of a serious illness that would later prove to be cancer. Although she had withdrawn from active participation in the affairs of the Woman's Hospital as she became ill, she nonetheless urged the Ladies' Board to accept the anonymous offer for the cancer pavilion—without knowing her cousin's involvement.

Eventually, Mrs. Astor told her cousin about her part in the offer, and the two of them, joined by her husband, John Jacob Astor III, began the plans for the New York Cancer Hospital.

John Jacob Astor III

There was an atmosphere of both hope and hopelessness when ground was broken in May 1884 for the new hospital, to be built as a state-of-the-art facility, with round towers to deter germs and keep dirt from accumulating in sharp corners and a vertical airshaft in each tower to prevent air from stagnating. A week after the cornerstone was laid, Mrs. Cullum died of cancer; a week after the hospital opened in December 1887, Mrs. Astor herself died of cancer.

Even after the hospital opened, little could convince people to shed the secrecy and seek medical care there before their cases were hopeless. In the four months prior to February 1894, four years after the hospital had opened, 81 percent of the patients admitted were inoperable or in such condition that surgery was useless. The patients, a staff member wrote, had operable cancers that "reach(ed) the surgeon too late to warrant expectation of cure." The hospital became known as "the Bastille," a place to be feared and avoided by both patients and patrons. In 1899, in an effort to attract more of both, administrators of the beleaguered hospital changed its name to the General Memorial Hospital. Years later, it would become known by a different name, Sloan-Kettering, and is now the Memorial Sloan-Kettering Cancer Center.

And though the cures were iffy and the treatment techniques crude—grafts of chicken skin when human skin was unavailable, poultices of flaxseed or balsam of pine, silver wire sutures or horsehair plucked from the horse at a nearby stable for the surgeries, whiskey for both sustenance and pain—prominent New York gynecologic surgeon Clement Cleveland and others who dealt daily with these deaths felt that so much more could be accomplished. "If only I'd been a year earlier, a month earlier, a week earlier, the outcome would have been different. It's as if the whole world seems to be in a conspiracy to turn cancer into something shameful," he told his young daughter, who would remember his words for the rest of her life.

Such thinking would prove to be visionary.

Cancer is at least as old as humanity itself. For many centuries, cancer was believed to be more prevalent in women than men because women were twice as likely to receive

Left: John Jacob Astor III married Charlotte Augusta Gibbes in 1846. When the Woman's Hospital, of which Augusta was a board member, refused to treat cancer patients, she convinced her husband to help finance the first wing of the New York Cancer Hospital, which was named Astor Pavilion in her honor. Right: Though once thought to be primarily a women's disease, autopsies and the use of the modern microscope revealed cancer to be responsible for many deaths in men as well.

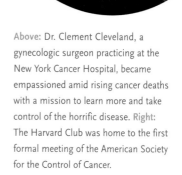

Above: Dr. Clement Cleveland, a gynecologic surgeon practicing at the New York Cancer Hospital, became empassioned amid rising cancer deaths with a mission to learn more and take control of the horrific disease. Right: The Harvard Club was home to the first formal meeting of the American Society for the Control of Cancer.

The American Cancer Society

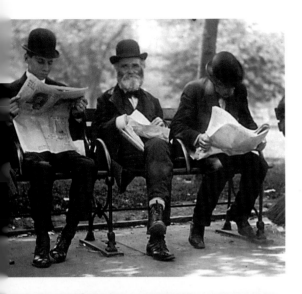

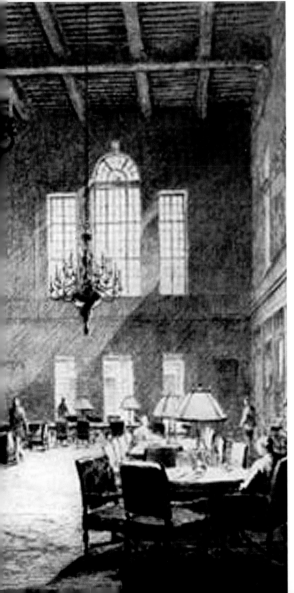

a cancer diagnosis. In the United States a deep-seated cultural fear of cancer as a major threat to men as well as women emerged during the second half of the nineteenth century, when doctors reported an alarming increase in cancer rates among men. Physicians put forward several reasons to account for this increase: medical advances, such as microscopic examination and more frequent autopsies, revealed many previously hidden cancers as the actual cause of death in men as well as women; a gradual increase in the life span of both men and women allowed more cancers to develop; and environmental factors, such as urbanization and the stress of modern life, might have weakened the body.

This growing knowledge, first collected at the New York Cancer Hospital, led Clement Cleveland and other physicians to see cancer as a significant problem not just for individuals, but for society. By 1912, a statistician with the Prudential Life Insurance Company reported what appeared to be a rapid increase in the incidence of cancer, moving in only a decade from the tenth most common cause of death in the United States to the fourth. Only infectious diseases like pneumonia, influenza, and tuberculosis were more deadly. When he reported this information in a presentation titled "The Menace of Cancer" at the 1913 meeting of the American Gynecological Society, physicians began to believe that the dissemination of known facts about cancer treatment and results could have an impact on both the public and the medical community.

Dr. Cleveland, sitting in the audience that day, was asked to pull together various groups interested in cancer education to begin developing a program for controlling the disease. The goal was to develop a national organization dedicated to the control of cancer. Representatives from the American Medical Association, the American Gynecological Society, the Clinical Congresses of Surgeons of North America (later to become the American College of Surgeons), the American Dermatological Association, and a number of prominent businessmen from New York trooped into the parlor of Dr. Cleveland's New York home. A month later, a formal meeting was held at the Harvard Club in New York.

In 1913, the American Society for the Control of Cancer, later to be known as the American Cancer Society, was formed. Its mission as a nationwide group was to gather facts and educate the public about cancer. Among the founding members were four physicians with direct ties to the New York Cancer Hospital and one woman.

That day, one of the founding members of the Society spoke prophetic words:

> *"We this morning are assisting in the inauguration of a moment . . . that will be of the greatest importance in the investigation of cancer."*

This is the story of how that prophecy came to be played out, carried into a new century by men and women of brave hearts, bright minds, and unrelenting dedication.

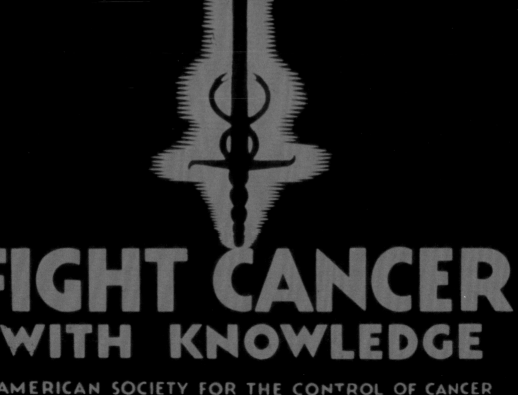

FIGHT CANCER
WITH KNOWLEDGE

AMERICAN SOCIETY FOR THE CONTROL OF CANCER

Fighting Cancer— with Knowledge

As studies go, it was a small one—only in Pennsylvania, only covering thirteen years, only a limited sampling. Yet, to physicians across the country, it was recording a seismic shift they were experiencing in their own medical practices.

The study, prepared by the Pennsylvania State Cancer Commission and published in 1924, traced the time it took cancer patients to seek care after they noticed symptoms that might be cancer—and, subsequently, the time it took doctors to offer treatment. The study showed that in Pennsylvania in 1910, patients with established cancers waited fourteen months on average to see a doctor after the first symptoms appeared. By the time they saw doctors, their cases were often so far advanced there was no hope. Yet thirteen years later, patients were visiting their doctors after only eight months—and were asking specific, cancer-related questions.

The study showed that the doctors themselves were changing the way they were practicing medicine. Although the medical community knew that there was a small percentage of doctors who were still dilatory and inefficient—the ones they called "the backward 10 percent"—most physicians were responding to their patients' new demands with more aggressive treatments. Doctors began to offer patients surgery to remove cancers—the only truly successful method of treatment at the time—almost 70 percent faster, assertively cutting the wait time from a full year in 1910 to just under four months in 1923.

The change was having a profound rippling effect on cancer treatment in the country. A doctor from St. Louis noted "a resulting slow but steady improvement in early diagnosis." Another at the Mayo Clinic in Minnesota declared, "Many cases have been cured as a result of early treatment." Patients, said a doctor from Wheeling, West Virginia, were "almost demanding information about cancer." And an Omaha doctor noted "a noticeable increase in the number of patients seeking advice" about cancer.

What, Doctors across America Puzzled, Was Going On?

As early as 1905, the American Medical Association (AMA) appointed a committee called the Council of Health and Public Instruction to examine the increase in cancer deaths. What they found was hardly reassuring. Most people in the United States at that time, including physicians, believed a cancer diagnosis was a death sentence and any action was useless. Many doctors were uninterested or unknowledgeable about treating cancer, routinely giving patients erroneous advice to "go home and forget it" or crediting symptoms to unlikely causes: bleeding from a cancerous uterus was ascribed to "rheumatism" or a "cold in the pelvis," while a man

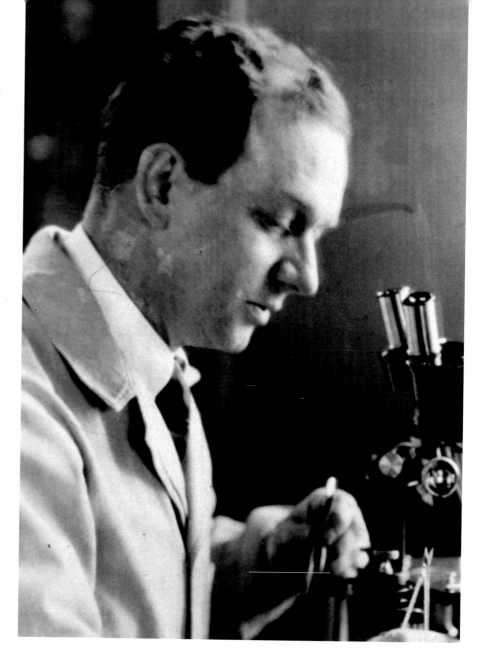

with rectal cancer was ordered "rest and a change of scenery."

Admittedly, a few things had happened on the cancer front in the years between 1910 and 1923 to cause this shift. In 1911, Peyton Rous, a young doctor two years out of medical school, identified a transmis-

"Tumors destroy man in a unique and appalling way, as flesh of his own flesh which has somehow been rendered proliferative, rampant, predatory, and ungovernable."

— Dr. Peyton Rous (above)

sible tumor virus in a Plymouth Rock hen, a discovery that began the journey from tumor virus biology to tumor biology itself, and would eventually lead to Dr. Rous receiving the Nobel Prize in 1966. In 1912, the Clinical Congresses of Surgeons of North America (now the American College of Surgeons) convinced a major women's magazine to run an article on cancer. And in 1915, cancer was induced in laboratory animals for the first time by a chemical—coal tar—applied to rabbit skin at Tokyo University. The lay public was getting into the act as well. The owner of a Montreal newspaper in 1922 offered one hundred thousand dollars to any graduate or student who could find the "medicinal treatment" for cancer within five years—and received more than three thousand claims of cures from forty different nations, four hundred of them from faith healers, herbalists, and fanatics. *Time* magazine, established in 1923, began routinely featuring articles on cancer under titles such as "Cancer Cure?" and "The Great Enigma."

Slowly, the taboo on the discussion of cancer that had hampered both research and treatment for a hundred years in the United States began to lift. From their patients, doctors were also seeing and hearing interesting things: talk of lectures and materials where descriptions of their symptoms were matter-of-factly described, pamphlets with names like *What You Should Know About Cancer* and *Fourteen Points About Cancer*.

This activity, the doctors began to acknowledge among themselves, was a result of the work of the American Society for the Control of Cancer (ASCC). "There can be no doubt that hundreds of lives . . . have been saved since the inception of the American Society for the Control of Cancer," said Dr. Frank W. Kenney of Denver in 1925. His comments, included in a slim, clothbound volume published by the Society that year to record its "objects and methods and some of the visible results of the work," were accompanied by almost two dozen others from doctors around the country. "It is apparent that both the physicians and the public at large are displaying an increased desire for information and an increased interest in the problems of cancer, for which condition I think it safe to assume the work of [the Society] is responsible," concluded Dr. Milton G. Sturgis of Seattle.

The Cancer Crusade had begun.

"Too damn clear"

The Society made it clear from its beginnings at the Harvard Club in New York City in May 1913 that it intended to fight cancer with information. Physicians estimated that

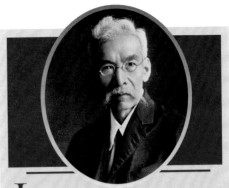

In 1915, Professor Katsusabura Yamagiwa, *above*, applied coal tar to rabbit ears every day for 660 days at Tokyo University. It marked the first time an experiment like this had been conducted in a laboratory setting. The rabbit ears, *left*, revealed squamous cell carcinoma from the repeated exposure to coal tar. These findings were predicted 140 years earlier by Percival Pott, *below*. Percival Pott was a surgeon at St. Bartholomew's Hospital in London from 1744 until 1787. He observed a high incidence of cancer in chimney sweeps and gardeners who had repeated exposure to burned coal residue. He was the first to establish a relationship between an occupation and cancer, becoming a pioneer in the science of epidemiology.

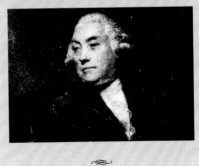

seventy-five thousand people were dying every year in America from cancer, and the numbers of deaths were skyrocketing in the early years of the twentieth century, as nearly a million immigrants arrived in the country annually.

In 1913, cancer was an enigma—seemingly resistant to the kinds of efforts that had begun to successfully control tuberculosis and pneumonia. Although physicians still believed it was spread by contagion, cancer didn't respond to sanitation or any of the methods commonly employed against infectious diseases. There seemed to be no drug or serum that could prevent or cure it. Dissemination of even the rudimentary information known was difficult, and treatment sometimes impossible.

The typical American medical school curriculum did not emphasize cancer diagnosis and treatment. Consequently, physicians graduated with little knowledge of the disease. As one early ASCC leader put it, "The cancer patient's fate was in the hands of the first physician they encountered," and those doctors all too often were neither knowledgeable nor eager to handle cancer patients.

In addition, physicians who practiced outside major metropolitan areas like New York City were frequently isolated and without access to the latest medical knowledge. Small-town doctors worked without diagnostic x-ray and laboratory studies, lacked modern pharmaceutical agents, often had no close colleagues with whom to exchange opinions, and were sometimes far away from hospitals.

Patients themselves didn't seek care

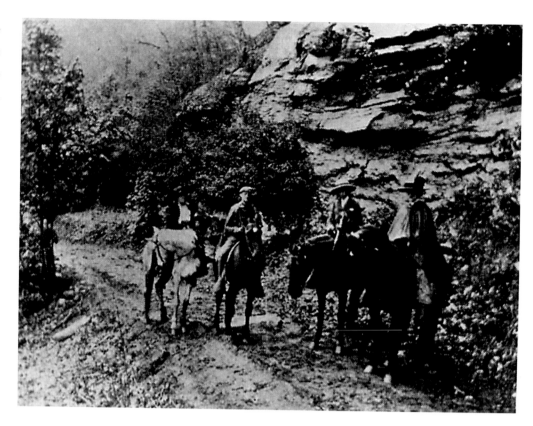

until they were desperate. They often treated themselves and alternately revered or feared their doctors and the medical treatments they prescribed. When patients did acknowledge their illnesses, the sick were often driven by desperation and ignorance to seek help outside accepted medical practices—giving strength to quacks and charlatans offering surefire "cures."

Yet there had already been hints for years of at least some surgical successes, if cancer cases were diagnosed early enough. A physician named William Stewart Halsted performed the first radical mastectomy in 1882 and stated in his accompanying paper that "more women could be cured with early diagnosis and treatment." In the same publication

Above: Three nurses, accompanied by a doctor, carefully pick their way along a treacherous road. Sick patients in rural areas such as this usually lacked ready access to health care and were often compelled by ignorance or desperation to accept any medical advice—including that offered by charlatans and quacks. **Opposite:** A new surgical amphitheatre at Johns Hopkins Hospital was formally opened on October 5, 1905. Dr. William Stewart Halsted (who two decades earlier had performed the first radical mastectomy) was persuaded by his staff to inaugurate the new facility by operating in it with all of his senior staff, rather than the usual residents—an event known as the "All-Star Operation." This operation took place early in the use of rubber gloves, a practice that began at Johns Hopkins.

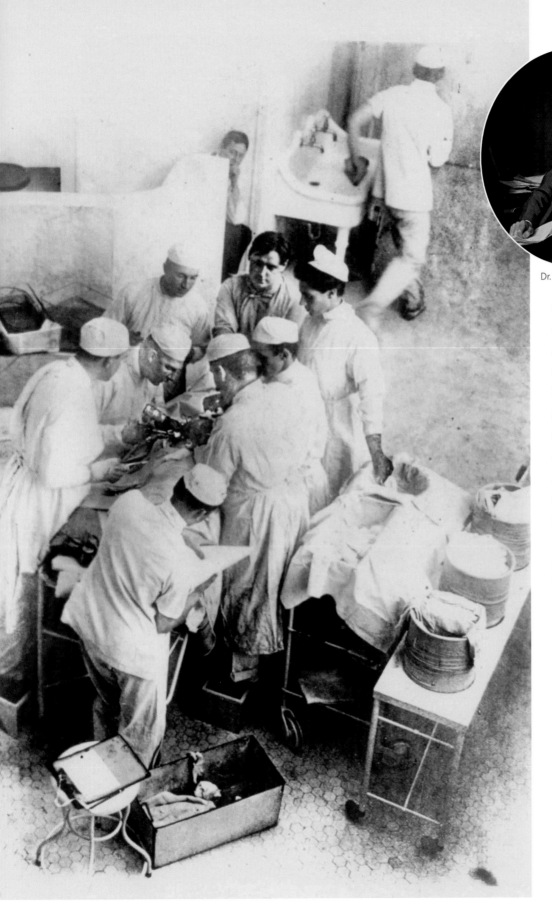

Dr. William Halsted

he posited that "both patients and referring physicians delayed referral out of a sense of hopelessness about curing the disease."

Two decades later, some European gynecologists were encouraging education of the public after successes with surgery in early-stage cervical cancer, and a few American doctors took note. As evidence mounted in the early 1900s, the rumblings to push public education grew louder from a few progressive surgeons and gynecologists. The AMA's 1905 cancer committee was the first attempt at this; this committee was joined in May 1912 by the American Gynecological Society (AGS), which devoted the entire third day of its annual meeting to a series of papers on the surgical treatment of cervical cancer. Each presentation pointed out the critical need for public education, and a committee of three physicians was named to gather suggestions and report their recommendations the following year to both the AGS and the AMA.

These efforts were all beginning to converge when a professor of gynecology at Johns Hopkins sat at his desk one October day in 1912, analyzing results of his cervical cancer cases to see how many patients were well after five years. Dr. Thomas S. Cullen found that only 23 percent of his patients were apparently still healthy. "I felt very blue about the situation," he wrote years later. "It was perfectly evident to me that if we were to get better results, it would be necessary to educate people as to the early symptoms of cancer."

Cullen wrote to the editor of a major medical publication about his concerns and was advised to bring up the issue at a meeting of surgeons in Brooklyn, New York, a month later. The idea of educating the public was readily adopted by the surgeons, many of whom knew of the AMA's own recommendations for more education, and a committee was formed to work on the issue, with Cullen as the chair. Cullen and his committee decided the best approach was to reach out to women. Not only was cancer still considered by many in the public to be a "woman's disease," but, as Cullen wrote, "it seemed wise to educate women . . . because, after all is said and done it is the wife, the mother, or the sister, who insists on a man going to the physician."

Cullen wrote a short article describing the signs and symptoms of uterine cancer and stressing the importance of early diagnosis and treatment. He hand-delivered it to the editor of the *Ladies' Home Journal*, one of the most popular women's magazines of the day. The editor, Karl Harriman, sat with a long black cigar while he read the article, puffing and scowling. Looking up from the paper, he finally told Cullen the article was "too damn clear; half our women readers would grab their hats and rush for the closest doctor." Instead, the editors at the *Journal* suggested a

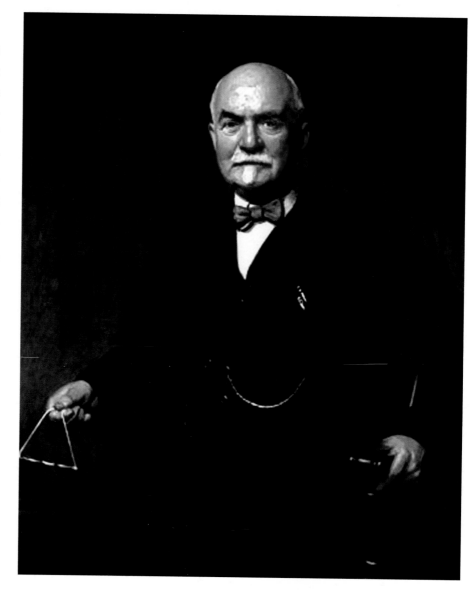

layperson should write the article—specifically, Samuel Hopkins Adams.

Adams was a crusading journalist whose articles often made a huge impact on the public. In 1905, he had written a series of eleven articles for *Collier's Weekly*, analyzing some of the country's most popular medicines, a series that led to the passing of the first Pure Food and Drugs Act the next year. Cullen invited

"It was perfectly evident to me that if we were to get better results, it would be necessary to educate people as to the early symptoms of cancer."

— Dr. Thomas S. Cullen (above)

What Can We Do About Cancer?

The Most Vital and Insistent Question in the Medical World

By Samuel Hopkins Adams

AUTHOR OF "THE GREAT AMERICAN FRAUD," ETC.

WHAT is to be done about cancer? No other question is so insistently demanding of medical science a definite reply. For some unascertained reason this dreaded scourge seems to be increasing in a startling ratio. A generation ago it was far down the list among the causes of death, not higher than tenth or twelfth. Today it ranks fifth or sixth: in some localities even as high as third, being exceeded in its number of victims only by tuberculosis and pneumonia. Latest comprehensive reports from England show that out of every eight women who attain the age of thirty-five years, one is slain by it; one out of every eleven men. In the year 1908 forty thousand Americans are known to have succumbed to it. General figures for the years since are not yet available, but local figures almost without exception indicate a startling growth. The next census may well show an appalling increase.

Notwithstanding this threatening condition no general movement has been, until recently, organized against the spread of the malady. Knowledge has lacked. Science has been face to face with a blank wall. Frankly and sadly it admits its fundamental ignorance.

Some fifteen years since I interviewed a number of physicians and surgeons on the question, "What causes cancer?" I received a wide variety of brilliant and conclusive answers, all of them wrong. In this year of enlightenment, 1913, I put the same query to a tableful of specialists, each with a nationwide reputation. One after another they made the

---

AN AUTHORITATIVE INDORSEMENT OF THIS ARTICLE

I HAVE read Mr. Adams's article on "What Can We Do About Cancer?" with the greatest interest. It gives in a most readable form the essence of our present knowledge on this subject. Surgeons are heartsick to see the many cancer patients begging for operations when the disease is so far advanced that nothing can be done.

Cancer is in the beginning a local process and not a blood disease, and in its early stages can be completely removed. When the cancer is small the surgeon can, with one-fourth the amount of labor, accomplish ten times the amount of good.

If the many readers of THE LADIES' HOME JOURNAL will profit by the advice given by Mr. Adams this article will be the means of saving thousands of lives.

THOMAS S. CULLEN, M.D.
Chairman of the Cancer Campaign Committee of the Congress of Surgeons of North America.

---

the mysteriously invading cell. It is known that no skin cancer ever develops except at a spot where there has been some previous and persistent irritation. There are curious proofs of this. Men who smoke clay pipes are peculiarly liable to cancer of the lip. This form is rare in women; where it occurs it usually develops that the woman is a smoker. Cancer of the tongue often arises from the slight chafing of a jagged tooth, the corollary to which is that a visit to the dentist may well be a life-saving move. In India the rough betel nut is carried all day in the hollow of the cheek by the natives. Cancer in India is most commonly found in the cheek; in Occidental countries it is almost unknown. Natives of Kurdistan, who go up into the cold mountain passes, wear a pan filled with live charcoal across the stomach. Among these people the prevalent location of cancer is on the skin of the abdomen, a spot practically exempt elsewhere in the world. "Chimney-sweep's cancer" is a well-recognized form. The sweep swings, while at his occupation, on a hard, narrow saddle, and the falling soot, trickling down his neck, irritates the skin at the point of pressure. Hence cancer of the groin is typical of the sooty brotherhood.

Any Irritation Should be Investigated at Once

BY ANALOGY it is inferred that internal cancers develop only after some prolonged irritation. Without this irritation they would not

---

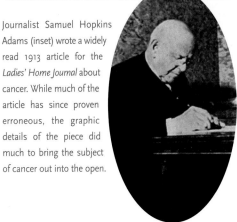

Journalist Samuel Hopkins Adams (inset) wrote a widely read 1913 article for the *Ladies' Home Journal* about cancer. While much of the article has since proven erroneous, the graphic details of the piece did much to bring the subject of cancer out into the open.

Adams to Baltimore for a dinner with some of the state's outstanding health leaders. They pumped Adams full of information about cancer, then sent him off to talk to doctors in Chicago and at the Mayo Clinic.

The two-page article Adams wrote, titled "What Can We Do About Cancer?" appeared in May 1913. Graphic and dramatic, much of the information the article provided was erroneous and primitive by today's knowledge, and it was accompanied by an endorsement from Cullen, as chair of the surgeons' cancer committee. Adams's reporting was picked up by other magazines and newspapers all over the country, with a combined estimated readership of eleven million. Cullen related that shortly after the article appeared, he met a surgeon from the South headed to an AMA meeting who told him, "Cullen, as a result of the *Ladies' Home Journal*

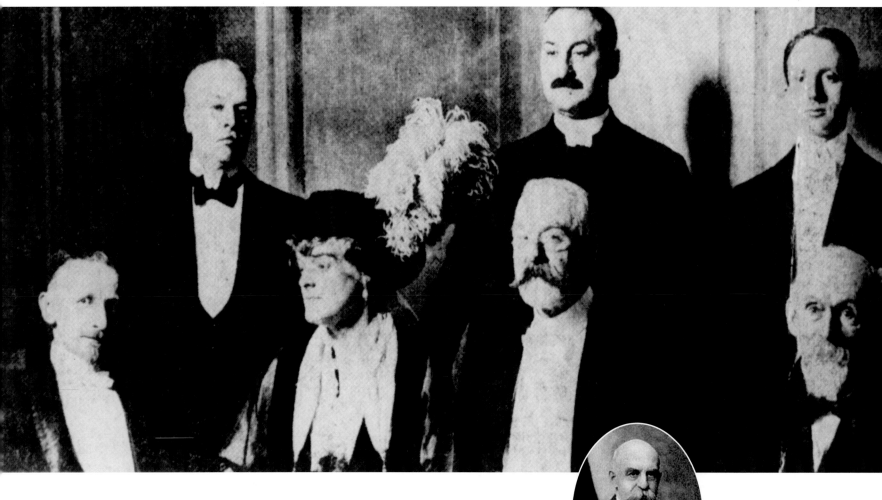

article, I have had six early cases of cancer in a little over a week."

On May 22, 1913, after a year of discussions and with the blessing and participation of more than two dozen medical groups, Dr. Clement Cleveland, nine other doctors, and five laypeople officially formed the American Society for the Control of Cancer. The organization was formed with two main goals: to gather information about cancer and to use that information to educate health care professionals and the public.

The Society's slogan was "Fight cancer with knowledge."

It was an incredible effort to undertake. The Society had no money and no structure. Medical professionals harbored a tremendous amount of skepticism that words—and words alone, since the first efforts of the Society did not include medical research of any sort, a path it did not veer from until 1946—could make any difference. And although it had been formed by doctors, the Society would rely heavily on both

Above: Seven of the original founders of the American Society for the Control of Cancer. Standing (left to right): Edward A. Woods; Rabbi J. Leonard Levy; Curtis E. Lakeman. Sitting (left to right): Dr. Frederick L. Hoffman; Mrs. Elsie Mead; Dr. Edward Reynolds; Dr. John A. Brashear. Inset: Dr. Clement Cleveland was also one of the founders of the American Society for the Control of Cancer. Opposite: Dr. Joseph C. Bloodgood, along with Dr. Thomas Cullen, advanced the frozen section technique of surgical pathology.

"The particular objects for which the corporation is to be formed are as follows: To collect, collate and disseminate information concerning the symptoms, diagnosis, treatment and prevention of cancer; to investigate the conditions under which cancer is found; and to compile statistics in regard thereto."

— Quote of the mission spelled out in the first certificate of incorporation, passed in 1922

LIKE MINDS

The American Society for the Control of Cancer began with the blessing of more than a dozen medical organizations. Present at the first meeting in May 1913 were representatives from the American Surgical Association, the American Gynecological Society, the American Association of Pathologists and Bacteriologists, the American Orthopedic Association, the American Ophthalmological Society, the American Neurological Association, the American Association of Genitourinary Surgeons, the American Otological Society, the American Laryngological Association, and the American Dermatological Association.

In addition, the American Medical Association, the American Surgical Association, the Clinical Congress of Surgeons, the Western Surgical Association, the Southern Surgical and Gynecological Association, the Southern Medical Association, the American Public Health Association, and many other national, state, and local medical societies endorsed the new Society and agreed to cooperate with it.

the generosity and leadership of laypeople—its first president was a New York stockbroker. The combination of laypeople and medical professionals was unprecedented and would both cause friction and instigate change for the Society.

For the Society, information was the key—to everything. Its objectives were both epidemiologic and educational. It wanted to act as a clearinghouse for the most modern medical information about cancer to be shared with both doctors and the public. On the medical front, the Society began to create a systematic and uniform record of cancer cases in hospitals and dispensaries in order to provide data on the value of surgical treatments—a forerunner of today's facts and figures about cancer. This approach in itself was revolutionary: no one kept statistics on cancer, because patients routinely begged their doctors to hide the diagnosis out of fear their families would be ostracized and because doctors often were either ignorant or uncertain about a cancer diagnosis.

Dr. Joseph C. Bloodgood

Raising Funds, Fueling Progress

The first lay leaders of the ASCC were all outstanding businesspeople from New York, and the first medical leaders were primarily from East Coast cities with established medical centers. One of the challenges of the Society was to reach beyond the large cities into more midsized and even smaller communities throughout the country. To make the Society a truly national effort, however, physicians from many universities and hospitals across the country were included on the first board, executive committee, and advisory council. Physicians were named as regional and state chairmen to represent the Society. The ASCC in some cases still depended on its founding core to be these chairpeople; among those first physician chairmen was Thomas Cullen, who cochaired the Maryland committee with Joseph C. Bloodgood. (The two men, both of Johns Hopkins Hospital, led the way toward origination and acceptance of the frozen section technique of surgical pathology.) But the Society also sought out doctors in Montana, Alabama, Idaho, Arkansas, Wyoming—anywhere that progressive doctors thought the work of the ASCC would make a difference.

In addition to complex organizational challenges, there was an immediate need to raise money to support the educational programs of the new Society. The original plan was to offer several categories of ASCC membership, depending on the level of donation.

Elsie Mead, a Society founder and daughter of Dr. Clement Cleveland, was named temporary head of the Ways and Means Committee, and she convinced five New York business leaders to guarantee one thousand dollars each toward the expenses for the first year. Mead then set about raising money from other sources. She interested a number of women of means in giving money to the Society and was so successful that she did not need to ask the original guarantors for their one thousand dollars.

~

The first permanent office space was rented in 1914 at 105 East 22nd Street in New York City, and a full-time secretary was hired. Now the national Society headquarters had an office, full-time staff, ongoing office expenses, and what seemed like a clear mission.

Playing on the success of the article a year earlier in the *Ladies' Home Journal*, the Society organized a series of town meetings, the first one held in Pittsburgh in February 1914, and subsequent others in New Orleans, Chicago, St. Louis, Boston, New York, and Portland, Maine. In each case, a panel of experts talked about symptoms and early diagnosis, stressing both what was known and what the ASCC thought could be done. Elsie Mead, recognizing that women might be reluctant to ask questions in such a public forum, approached the General Federation of Women's Clubs and asked them to help her organize a series of small "parlor meetings" on

cancer in other communities. The collaboration with the national women's clubs would prove incredibly helpful to the Society in later years (see Chapter 2, "Women's Influence").

By 1922, the Society had an office, a staff, program and materials costs, and a presence in all forty-eight states and three provinces in Canada. With increased demand for services and rising materials costs, however, money was becoming tight, and the Society turned to its board of directors and executive committee for help. Each member pledged one hundred dollars to pay the Society's expenses for that year. The original financial plan for the American Society for

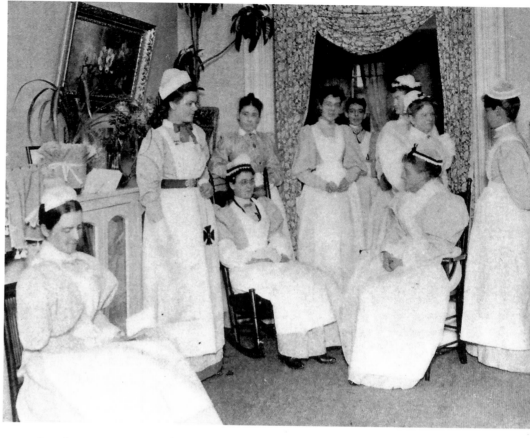

Above: Members of a club for nurses that was affiliated with the General Federation of Women's Clubs and formed in New York in 1894. Opposite: Early publications of the American Society for the Control of Cancer. Published in 1914, *The Story of Mrs. Harrison* told the tale of a woman cured of breast cancer and concludes with the words, "IN THE EARLY TREATMENT OF CANCER LIES THE HOPE OF CURE." Opposite inset: Dr. Charles Powers, president of the ASCC in 1919, pioneered the use of radio to spread the word about cancer, stressing early diagnosis.

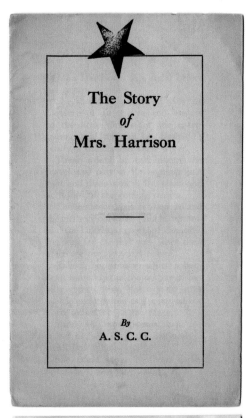

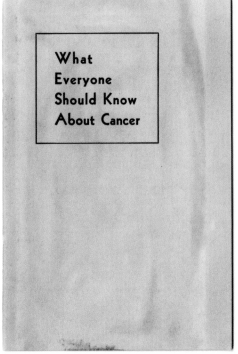

the Control of Cancer called for the national office of the Society to raise its money and each of the Division offices to conduct independent fundraising activities. There was to be no intermingling of funds between the national office and geographic divisions of the Society. That system lasted until 1922, when the board of directors of the national ASCC voted to request that Divisions provide financial support to the national office. The amount of money to be sent to national would be based on a formula, using the population and per-capita income of each state.

The increasing work of the ASCC was reflected in its annual budgets. The cost of running the Society averaged between five thousand and nine thousand dollars for the early years 1914 to 1919, inclusive. In 1920, with the first world war behind the nation and the Society's work expanded, expenses increased by more than 50 percent. In the next year, they nearly doubled; by 1924, the Society was spending almost forty-seven thousand dollars annually. The new push in outreach resulted in an 800 percent increased demand for cancer education pamphlets and booklets. People everywhere, particularly women, were becoming accustomed to hearing and reading about cancer. The *Ladies' Home Journal* again published a short article on cancer, and nurses throughout the country were being asked to help fight cancer by stressing the need for early treatment. State and county medical societies were linking

arms with the ASCC, and the National Safety Council circulated six million bulletins on cancer to workers throughout the country.

Taking Up the Sword

The Society's National Home Office developed a lending library of cancer publications, and in 1919 the first sets of teaching medical lantern slides about cancer were produced and made available to physicians and the public for cancer education. In 1920, the Society designed and sponsored a public exhibit and placed it in the American Museum of Natural History in New York City. The exhibits graphically displayed the signs and symptoms of common cancers and emphasized the importance of early diagnosis and proper treatment. In 1921, with a grant from the Laura Spelman Rockefeller Memorial, the first cancer education–themed motion picture was produced, titled *The Reward of Courage*.

But the Society knew it needed additional ways to focus America's attention on the cancer problem, and in 1921 it sponsored its first National Cancer Week. Copies of *The Reward of Courage* were distributed nationwide. A number of articles also appeared in popular women's magazines. Educational programs were held in every state, and it was estimated that more than five hundred thousand people received lifesaving information about cancer. Dr. Charles Powers, who had been elected president of the Society in 1919, for the first time

Dr. Charles Powers

used the national radio media to broadcast messages about cancer, stressing the importance of early diagnosis and treatment.

The melding of national, regional, and grassroots components was a harbinger of today's American Cancer Society, and it struck a chord that still resonates today. The second National Cancer Week a year later made use of two thousand volunteers across the country to distribute information and was accompanied by an endorsement from the White House. Interestingly, President Warren G. Harding's endorsement letter never mentioned the word "cancer." The letter stated: "Concerning this particular disease . . . I hope that the effort you are making to create a proper public understanding of the whole subject will be marked by a great success along those lines. . . . No single misfortune of the race has so sharply challenged science." The omission of the word "cancer" reflects the social stigma that continued to be associated with the disease.

The response of some in the medical profession to National Cancer Week was less than enthusiastic. Was there a move toward too much information? Some felt, as an article in the *Journal of the American Medical Association* editorialized in 1921, "an inevitable accompaniment of directing special attention to any disease is to arouse . . . phobias almost as terrifying as the disease feared."

Dr. George A. Soper

Even some of the Society's own questioned its methods. Dr. George A. Soper, hired by the Society as its first managing director in 1923, suggested it was "questionable whether the optimistic attitude [that ASCC materials emphasized] furnishes the strongest motive force." Should the ASCC be relentlessly optimistic, or should it motivate through fear?

The medical industry was very sensitive to any educational efforts aimed at laypeople, and the Society's efforts were not always delicate enough to avoid giving offense. There was also a question of exactly how much impact the ASCC was having. Despite the glowing numbers and endorsements from the 1924 Pennsylvania report, a survey done in 1927 by an ASCC field representative—a position created in 1922—brought discouraging news. There were no cancer hospitals or clinics in Texas; the Washington state chairman had resigned because he believed the Society was creating "undue alarm"; and cancer deaths in Montana rose from forty per one thousand in 1910 to seventy-nine per one thousand in 1926.

Yet the world was catching on to the potential for success through the Society, and funds were starting to come in to support its work. In 1923, the American Society for the Control of Cancer was legally incorporated

Left: Dr. George A. Soper was hired in 1923 as the first managing director of the Society. Opposite: A free Cancer Prevention Detection Center in Brooklyn, New York, was one more way to encourage citizens to get an early diagnosis.

in New York state. This legal process codified the relationship between the national organization and the Divisions and clearly spelled out a formula for revenue sharing. A second reason for incorporating the Society was to enable the ASCC to receive major donations and bequests as a New York charitable institution.

The Society's leadership was moving in ever-higher circles and reaping the benefits of its connections and its work. In 1926, the ASCC received a gift of two hundred fifty thousand dollars from John D. Rockefeller to support its cancer control activities. Mirroring an earlier effort by a Montreal newspaper owner, the head of a major manufacturing company offered a prize of one hundred thousand dollars in 1926 for the first researcher to find a cure for cancer.

In 1927, the Society developed a plan to raise a million dollars as an endowment. A leading New York financier and philanthropist named R. Fulton Cutting, who later became president of the Cooper Union, offered a two hundred fifty thousand dollar memorial to his wife as a challenge to the Society to raise the remaining seven hundred fifty thousand dollars. Elsie Mead accepted the challenge and through a series of special events helped the Society meet its goal.

Clearly, the war on cancer required more than pamphlets and speakers. The public and its medical leaders both needed up-to-date information on cancer. Soper, an

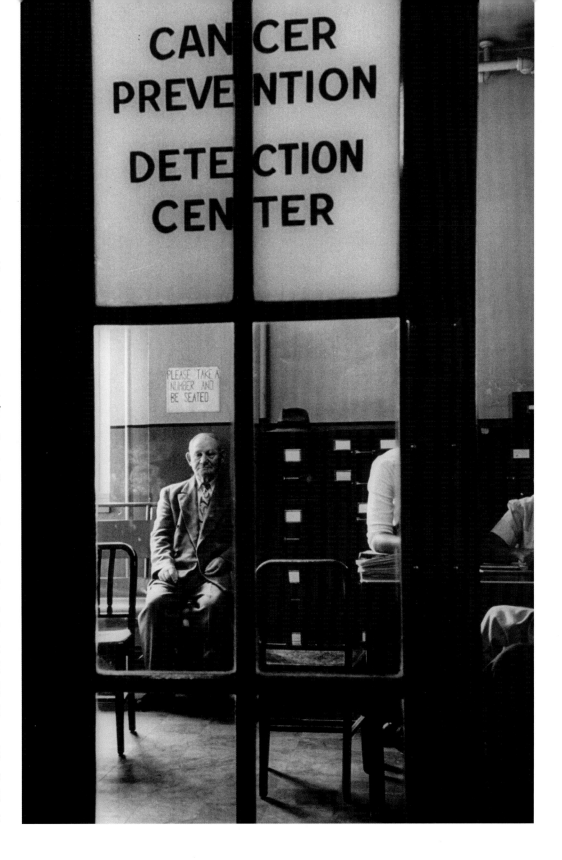

epidemiologist who had helped track down "Typhoid Mary," the first healthy carrier of that disease in the United States, began to push the Society to collect better data. To do so, he turned to a model being tried by a Boston surgeon named Dr. Ernest Codman. Dr. Codman had developed a cancer registry for the purpose of determining the cure rate of patients with bone tumors, evaluating treatment through long-term follow-up with patients over a number of years. Soper believed the ASCC could emulate Codman by supporting fact-gathering efforts and increasing treatment success through a series of cancer clinics around the United States. By 1926, three years after Soper became managing director of the Society, there were fifteen cancer clinics in the country—still a far cry from the eight hundred venereal disease clinics, six hundred tuberculosis clinics, and more than one hundred heart clinics, but a start nonetheless. Supporting the clinics became a major project of the Society, and by 1930 there were more than two hundred fifty cancer clinics sponsored by the ASCC nationwide.

Along with diagnosis and treatment, the clinics developed programs for gathering epidemiologic information, registering cancer patients, and following them for years to determine treatment outcomes. In later years, the American College of Surgeons developed standards for the clinics, in cooperation with the ASCC, and required each of the clinics to contribute data to a cancer tumor registry. Over the years, these clinics and their registries

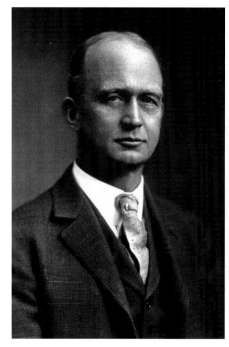

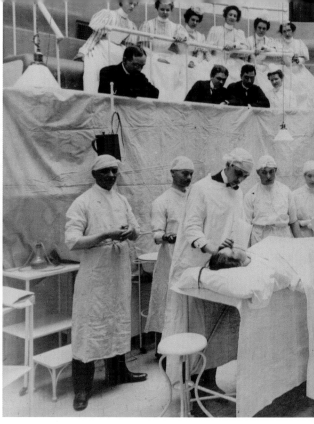

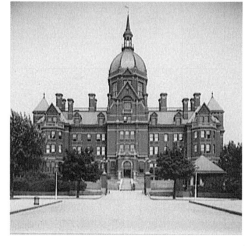

Above: In an effort to collect better data about cancer, the Society turned to a cancer registry model developed by Dr. Ernest Codman of Boston. **Right and opposite:** By the 1920s and 1930s, cancer programs began to proliferate at hospitals around the country. Hospital of the Good Shepherd (above); American Oncologic Hospital (upper right); Johns Hopkins Hospital in Maryland (bottom left); St. Luke's Hospital (bottom center); and Garfield Hospital (bottom right).

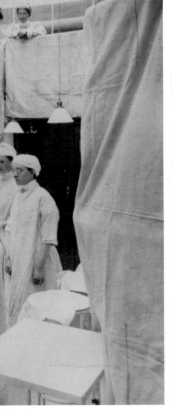

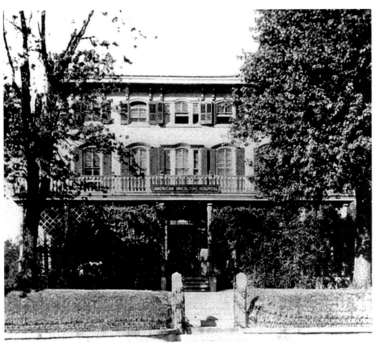

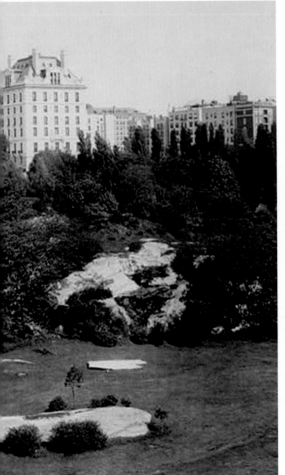

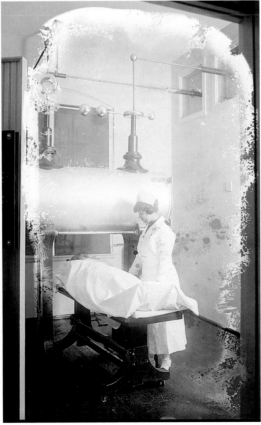

A Close Connection

The ASCC and the American College of Surgeons have been intertwined almost since the beginning of both organizations. Both were formed in May 1913 a few days apart, and many founding members of the surgical group became members of the ASCC.

When the ASCC decided it needed a way to certify its cancer clinics, it turned to the surgeons' group. The goal of the clinics was to improve the quality of diagnosis and treatment of suspected cancer patients. The Society's medical field officer was assigned to monitor the clinics. As the number of clinics increased, the logistics became impossible: at one point, the Society even discussed buying an airplane so that the field officers could shuttle from clinic to clinic.

The solution came in 1930 with a grant from the ASCC to the American College of Surgeons to develop standards for cancer clinics and to regularly survey each clinic on site. The program would eventually come to be known as the Approved Hospital Cancer Program of the American College of Surgeons.

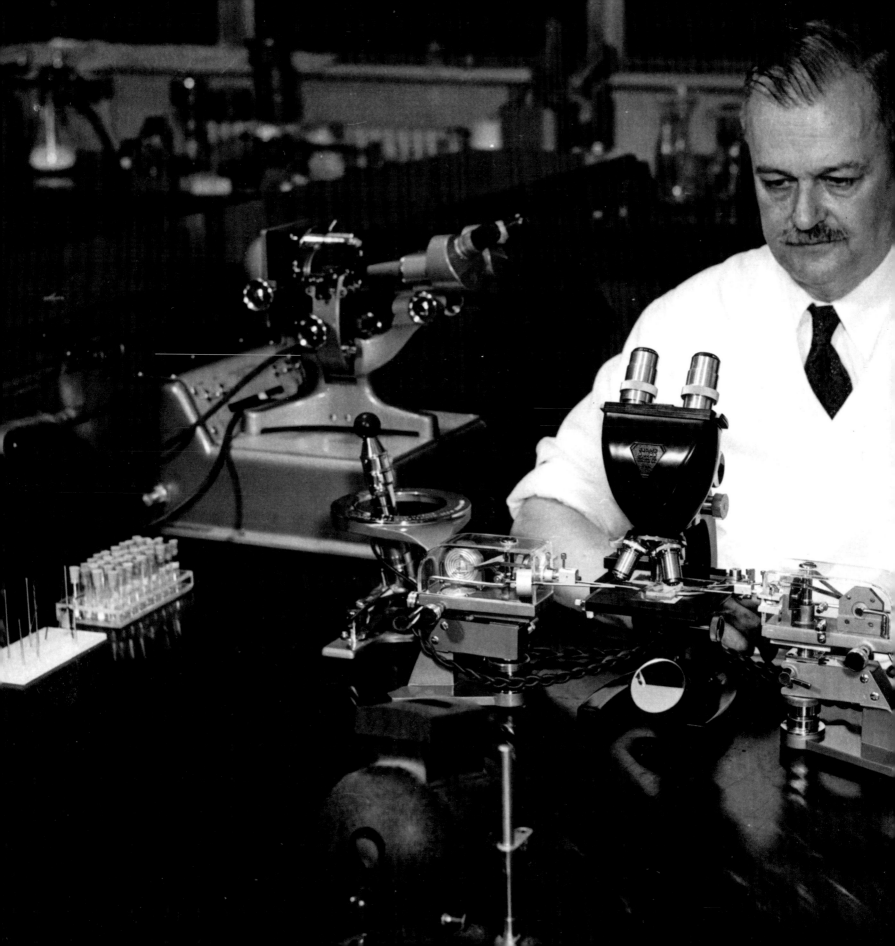

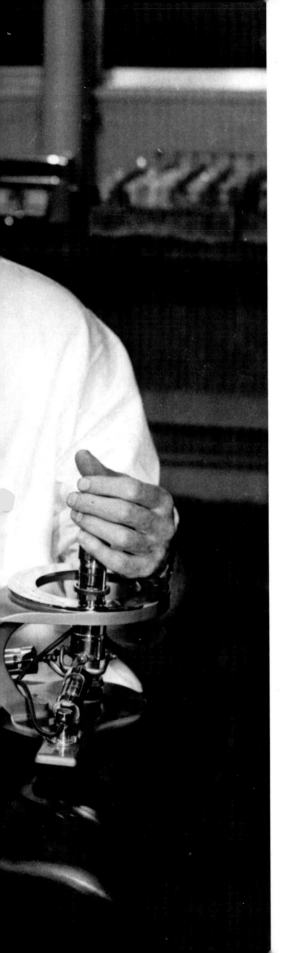

evolved into the hospital cancer programs of the Approved Hospital Cancer Program of the American College of Surgeons. Today, there are approximately fifteen hundred Commission on Cancer–approved cancer programs in the United States, which diagnose and treat the majority of the cancer patients in the country.

A Growing Outreach

Years of work were paying some dividends, but the Society needed more volunteers and funding to support its programs. Its almost totally male leadership—top-heavy with physicians and scientists still tied to a handful of East Coast communities, dominated by New York City—was constraining its work. Twenty years after its founding, there was still a schism between the Society and the medical industry about the effectiveness of its work in educating the public. Dr. Clarence Cook Little, named managing director of the Society in 1929 to replace Soper, visited Europe in 1930 to meet with health professionals there. He found they were almost unanimously opposed to lay education in cancer, because of the fear of creating cancer phobia.

The ASCC, however, was determined to press on with its mission to educate the public, both lay and medical. To do so, Little would tap into a segment of society that was sixty million strong and who a century later would make up 75 percent of the Society's volunteer workforce—women.

Little recognized two simple truths, the same ones Thomas Cullen had acknowledged when he went to the *Ladies' Home Journal* to get the first cancer article published: Women accounted for a large portion of recorded cancer cases, and they had a great deal of influence over when and from whom their families sought medical care. And, although small in numbers, they had been a part of the ASCC since its inception and part of the fight against cancer for even longer. Women's influence would bring what a future Society leader—and its first woman board chair—called "the weight of gold" to the efforts to cure cancer.

❧

"Why do I feel so deeply about it? . . . Because my own father died as a result of cancer. Because perhaps whatever ancestral desire I have to explore the unknown is appealed to by the research work and the wish to be a 'crusader,' which almost all of us have, is given a chance to express itself. Finally, because I believe that Americans will be happier and saner if they combine in fighting a scourge like cancer than they will be if they continue to fight each other for money and power."

— Dr. Clarence Cook Little
Time magazine, March 22, 1937

❧

Left: Dr. Clarence Cook Little in his laboratory

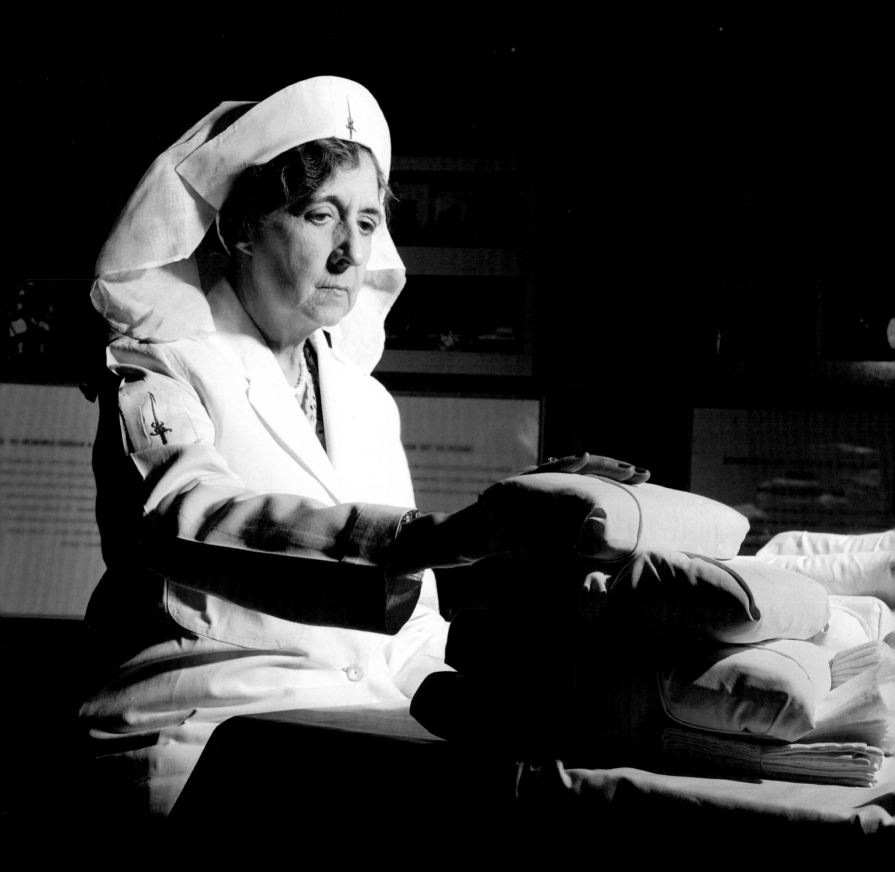

Women's Influence

Dr. Clarence Cook Little lived in a world of mice and men. And, while both were huge contributors to the fight against cancer, he had come to the conclusion that neither could supply him with what he desperately needed for the American Society for the Control of Cancer: grassroots strength and financial support.

Little was a scientist and a member of an old Boston family descended from Paul Revere. His boyhood was spent on the family estate just outside Boston amid a variety of pets, including his own squeaking mice and pedigreed pigeons. He was a Harvard man, the captain of the track team, a handsome and outgoing raconteur who, by the time he came to the ASCC in 1929 as its managing director,

Left: A volunteer in the Women's Field Army

had been the youngest college president ever in the country at the University of Maine and served a tumultuous four-year term as president at the University of Michigan.

Throughout all this, he continued studying the new science of mammalian genetics, including its intersection with cancer. He had become fascinated with the cancer problem while at Harvard and began to raise mice in order to study genetics and tumors. Eventually, he created two highly useful inbred strains of mice that would prove crucial to his cancer research.

While research was his first love, it was expensive. When he accepted his second college presidency in the mid-1920s, Little

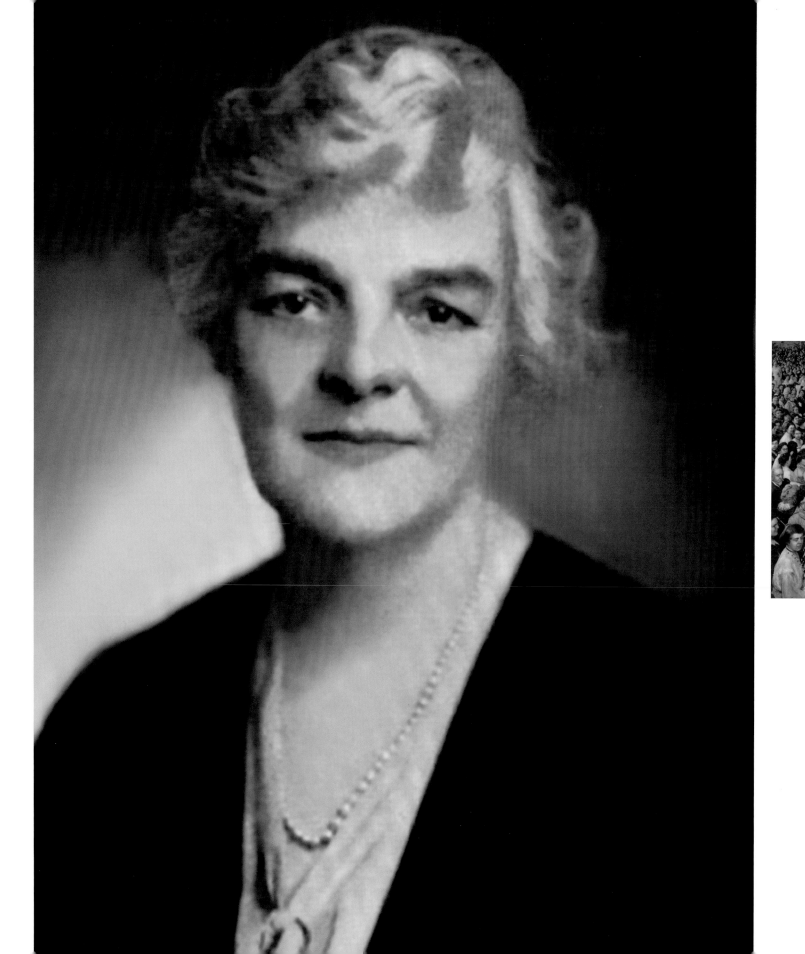

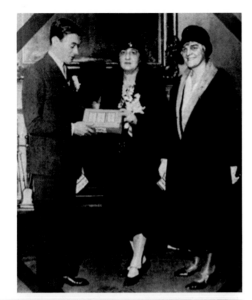

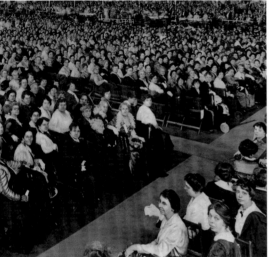

Opposite: Elsie Mead, chairman of the Society's Ways and Means Committee, worked closely with the General Federation of Women's Clubs in order to get access to the federation's two million members. Mead worked tirelessly, even going to her wealthy friends, to help keep the cash-strapped Society afloat. Top: Elsie Mead in 1928, accompanied by New York City Mayor Jimmy Walker and Mrs. Samuel Adams Clark, one of the early leaders of the New York City Cancer Committee. The photo was taken at the first fundraising campaign for the Society. Above: The thirteenth biennial convention of the General Federation of Women's Clubs. Above right: Dr. Clarence Cook Little, a Harvard-educated scientist and raconteur, was one of the country's leading cancer researchers and later managing director of the Society.

negotiated what was then an unprecedented five thousand dollars for research assistance. In 1929, he'd once again accepted a dual challenge: he'd started the Roscoe B. Jackson Memorial Laboratory in Bar Harbor, Maine, to raise his mice and study cancer, and he'd agreed to become managing director of the ASCC. Again, needs were overlapping: both his laboratory and the Society needed an influx of funds.

From the early days of the ASCC, women's organizations played a pivotal role in the dissemination of the messages and materials of the Society. This collaboration and partnership began in 1913 with a close association between Elsie Mead, chairman of the Ways and Means Committee of the ASCC, and Grace Morrison Reynolds, the national president of the General Federation of Women's Clubs. The federation was one of the oldest and largest women's groups in America, with two million members. At Mead's request, hundreds of member clubs had sponsored regular "parlor meetings" during the Society's early years, educating women about cancer and distributing the messages of the ASCC throughout the United States.

Yet women were still very much on the sidelines of the Society. Mead was a rare female presence in the world of male doctors, scientists, and the very few lay members who made up the Society. Although women were often inspirational and effective as organizers of social reform groups—Clara Barton founded the American Red Cross, seven women and one man established the American branch of the Salvation Army, a nineteen-year-old woman from a prominent family began the Junior League—most were neither trained nor allowed to take on management roles outside the home.

Dr. Clarence Cook Little

Women were, however, extremely effective fundraisers. Elsie Mead almost single-handedly kept the Society bankrolled for twenty years, calling on her women society friends to help keep the cash-strapped organization afloat, once raising seven hundred fifty thousand dollars in a single year, an unprecedented amount in the 1920s.

Little took over the top staff position of the ASCC just before the 1929 stock market crash that plunged the nation into the Great Depression. He assumed control of an organization still unsure of its direction, and—not incidentally—completely male dominated. The male part was an issue because, as Dr. Thomas Cullen had pointed out years before when he sought to publish the first article about cancer in a magazine, it was "the women [who] . . . insist on a man going to the physician." Little already knew what women could accomplish. When he'd started his laboratory in Bar Harbor, he had hired six young men and one extraordinary woman, Elizabeth "Tibby" Russell, a brilliant scientist whose solid five-foot two-inch frame was packed with strut and principle. Russell got things done, and she was always the one in the room who asked the best questions. Little had also spent World War I in the Signal Corps, later to become the U.S. Air Force. Discharged in 1918 with the rank of major, he fully understood the power of military organization.

It would take a few years for Little to link together the need for money, the power of women, and the lure of the military. When he did, it would be a cataclysmic shift for the ASCC and its future as a volunteer-led, grassroots organization.

"Thousands . . . share the burden"

When Little first came to work for the ASCC in 1929, he believed the Society had devoted enough attention to lay education and too little to education for doctors and other medical professionals. He had heard only too well the concern in the medical community that the Society was whipping up paranoia and fear—and even offering false hope—with its educational materials, movies, and pamphlets, and the annual Cancer Weeks (see page 57) that

were now part of its public relations efforts. One of his first moves after arriving at the Society in 1929 was to divide the country into four geographic quadrants and hire four physicians to focus on professional education. He also wanted more emphasis on gathering epidemiologic information, which he believed was the way to determine where and how best to attack cancer.

By 1935, however, six years into his time with the Society, Little was seeing signs that the tide had turned too far. He was now convinced that public education was lagging behind professional development. Convincing others, and making it happen, however, was an uphill battle. Like other organizations, the ASCC had been hard-hit by the Great Depression. Money and volunteers, particularly the people he needed to make a big educational push, were gone.

Cancer wasn't.

The numbers were staggering. Cancer was now the number-two cause of death in America, behind infectious diseases. In 1937, there were three hundred thousand women in the United States with cancer. Eighty thousand of them would die that year of the disease. The ASCC believed forty thousand women could have been saved, had they been diagnosed and treated early enough. The fight against cancer was clearly stalled, and the American public wanted action.

Women, money, and the military were about to triangulate.

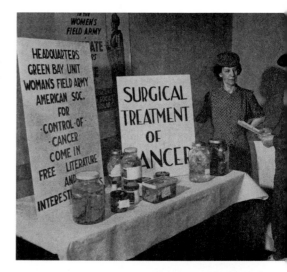

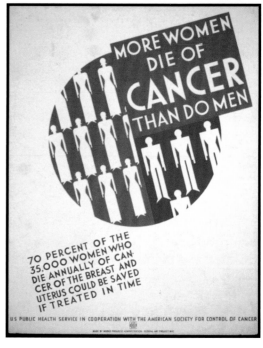

"Cancer kills 1 woman in 8 after 40."
— Dr. J. A. Gannon
American Society for the Control of Cancer
Washington Post, Nov. 2, 1921

Dr. Thomas Cullen

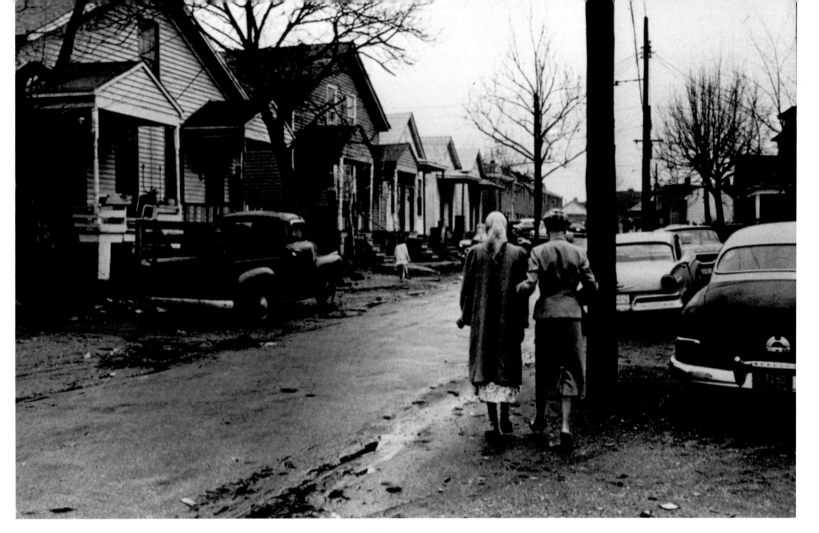

Opposite left inset: Dr. Thomas Cullen, a professor of gynecology, pushed for early detection education about cancer when he uncovered statistics that showed only 23 percent of women were still healthy five years after cancer treatment. Opposite top: An educational exhibit sponsored by the Green Bay, Wisconsin, Unit of the Women's Field Army. Above: A Women's Field Army volunteer helping a cancer patient in Tennessee. Launched in 1936, the Women's Field Army was a nationwide grassroots organization dedicated to assisting and educating people about cancer. Opposite bottom: A poster encouraging women to seek treatment for cancer, created as part of the Works Progress Administration Federal Art Project

Little had been working closely with the Federation of Women's Clubs since 1932, when he and the board officially enlisted their members in an underfunded public education campaign. Mrs. Marjorie Illig, chairman of the General Federation of Women's Clubs Committee on Public Health, was appointed lay field representative for the ASCC in 1936. Working together, Little and Illig prepared a proposal to involve clubwomen in the Society through a new "army" of volunteers. Little went to Dr. George H. Bigelow, ASCC president, with their idea to form an auxiliary organization that he wanted to call the Women's Field Army. Little and Illig saw this as a way to create a huge grassroots group, able to raise funds to wage "a great fight."

It took some convincing to bring the board along with the idea. Most of the board members were physicians, and they viewed cancer primarily as a medical problem to be dealt with by professionals. They controlled the board and sometimes viewed lay members as offering more annoyance than help; the idea of introducing more lay influence, and especially women, concerned some. But others saw the need to involve many different talents and types of expertise in the fight against cancer.

Cancer was too important to leave only to the physicians. Little wanted nothing less than a "widespread and intensive campaign" to inform the public about "the prevention of cancer," and he persuaded the board that the Women's Field Army was a way to do this. In 1936, with the full blessing of the ASCC board, Little created the Women's Field Army (WFA).

The Society also wanted action at the federal level: they wanted research money and attention paid to finding a cure for cancer. In 1937, they got just that, when the National Cancer Institute Act "boiled up spontaneously and nearly simultaneously" out of both the U.S. House and Senate, as one historian put it. The Society and the newly formed Women's Field Army threw its weight behind the bill. Although the American Medical Association opposed the bill because it worried, as the *Journal of the American Medical Association* put it, about the danger of letting government be "in a dominant position in . . . medical research," the bill was passionately supported by the American public, both men and women. The National Cancer Institute was created in 1937 as an independent research institute.

Little was featured in a *Time* magazine article five months before President Franklin D. Roosevelt signed the bill, proclaiming, "There is no longer a need to fight cancer alone. Hundreds of thousands will share the burden." He had already mobilized his "army" in the effort to get the Cancer Act passed; in its first year of existence, the Women's Field Army

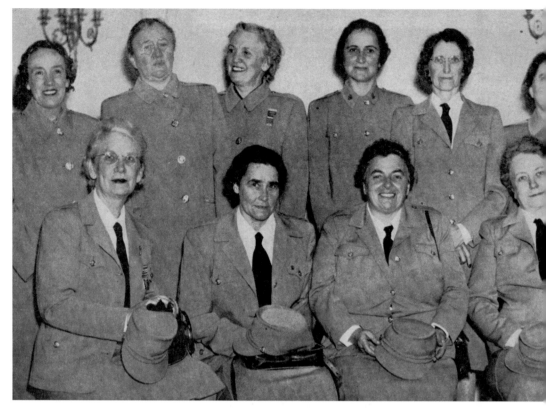

enlisted fifteen hundred women volunteers. And now he saw this group as a powerful tool in the ASCC arsenal. Not coincidentally, one of those thousands he cited who would share the burden was First Lady Eleanor Roosevelt, whom Little persuaded in 1938 to be the honorary chair of the Women's Field Army. A few years after the WFA's founding, Little was able to brag, "In 1935 there were fifteen thousand people active in cancer control throughout the United States. At the close of 1938, there were ten times that number."

The grassroots power of the Women's Field Army was tremendous. At its peak, it had seven hundred thousand dues-paying members, each paying a one-dollar enrollment

Above: Regional Commanders of the Women's Field Army, American Society for the Control of Cancer, 1942. Seated (left to right): Mrs. H. C. Peterson, Montana; Mrs. J. C. Carmack, Rhode Island; Mrs. Marjorie Illig, national commander, New York City; Mrs. H. B. Ritchie, Georgia. Standing (left to right): Mrs. Volney Taylor, Texas; Mrs. Harry W. Smith, New Hampshire; Mrs. David S. Long, Missouri; Mrs. Hobart Herbert, Tennessee; Mrs. Emily G. Bogert, Colorado; Mrs. John S. Harvey, West Virginia. Bottom: Dedication of the National Cancer Institute, which was formed in 1937 as a partially federally funded research organization.

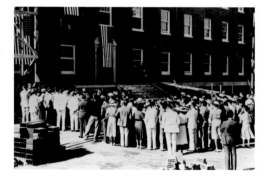

fee. Along with its own volunteers, it had a potential workforce of the two million members of the General Federation of Women's Clubs. It acted much like a military organization, with a national advisory board, regional and state commanders, area captains, local lieutenants, and members. The slogan of the WFA was the same as the ASCC, "Fight Cancer with Knowledge." The women's uniforms, designed by New York fashion designer Lilly Daché, echoed the mood of a country coming off one world war and headed into another. One physician, acknowledging the need for the organization, wrote, "When the dead and dying from cancer are regarded in a similar light to the slain and wounded on the field of battle . . . the same compulsion that leads to victory against an invading army will operate in the struggle to vanquish this disease." It was a very hands-on movement; the Women's Field Army developed programs that had a direct impact on cancer patients' quality of life. The WFA started a program to provide

Certificate of Enlistment

THIS CERTIFIES THAT

ENLISTED NAME   TOWN
IS A MEMBER OF THE GEORGIA DIVISION

WOMEN'S FIELD ARMY

AMERICAN SOCIETY FOR THE CONTROL OF CANCER, INC.

STATE COMMANDER   NATIONAL COMMANDER

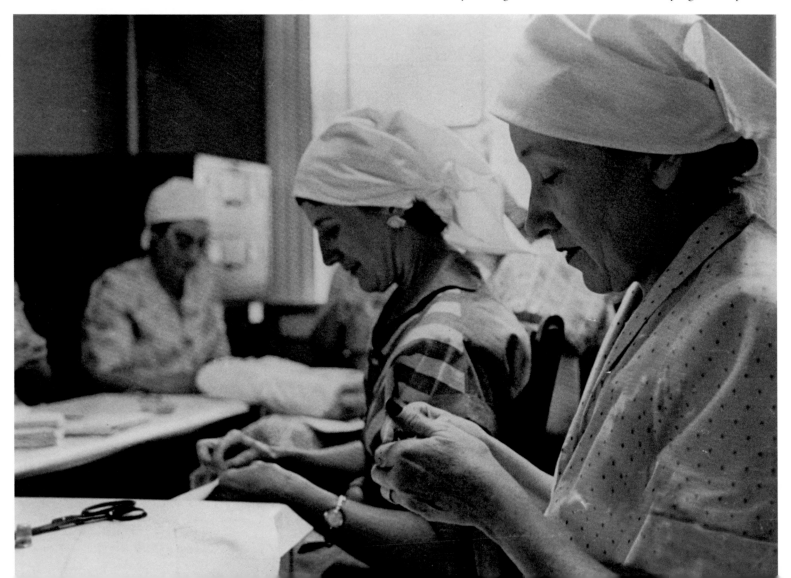

bandages and dressings to cancer patients; arranged transportation for those needing to go to doctors and hospitals; opened loan and gift closets that stocked sickroom equipment, linens, and the like; and staffed cancer clinics and information centers. The women were tremendous in their efforts to raise awareness—they distributed two million pieces of literature in 1943 alone and raised almost all the money supporting the Society for nearly a decade. Their numbers and innovative methods also helped move the Society to the forefront of voluntary health organizations.

In later years, Kathleen J. Horsch, who became the Society's first woman board chair in 1988, would praise the work of these women and those who followed. "Women were carrying forward the role of raising the dollars, public education, and transportation. Women were collectively driving the mission of the Society and its various programs. We really were the field army—the power and might of the effort."

At the same time, the Women's Field Army's growing strength was creating a rift within the Society. Two essentially separate cancer organizations were beginning to evolve, with overlapping goals and competing fundraising programs, one run by men, one by women, who still had no representation on the Society's board.

The divide became untenable and uncomfortable. Little began campaigning as early as 1941 for a complete reorganization, warning the board that pressure was coming

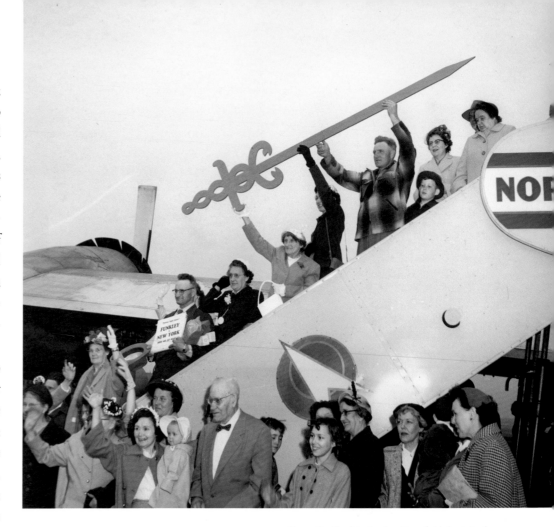

from the thousands of patients newly educated by the Society. If they couldn't get what they wanted from the Society, he said, the public would get it from some other organization. In other words, if the doctors wouldn't share power, they stood a good chance of losing it to some other cancer-control organization.

The physicians were still slow to respond, but in the end it hardly mattered. Another powerful woman named Mary Lasker was about to enter the picture and, in a quick, dramatic move, force a reorganization that would literally change the face of the ASCC.

Above: To stimulate the donation of old sheets to the Society's dressings program, the entire town of Funkley, Minnesota, was flown to New York City where they spent a week sightseeing. Every woman in the town of Funkley was enrolled in the cancer dressings program. Here "Funkleyites" arrive by plane at LaGuardia Airport.
Opposite top: Mary Lasker was wealthy and intelligent and led the effort, along with her husband, Albert (right), to increase funding for the fight against cancer.

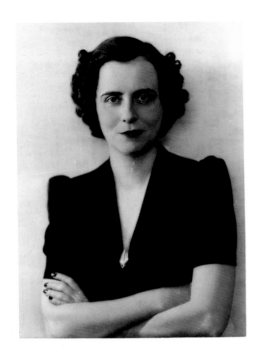

"Women were carrying forward the role of raising the dollars, public education, and transportation. Women were collectively driving the mission of the Society and its various programs. We really were the field army—the power and might of the effort."

— Kathleen J. Horsch
First woman board chair of the Society, 1988

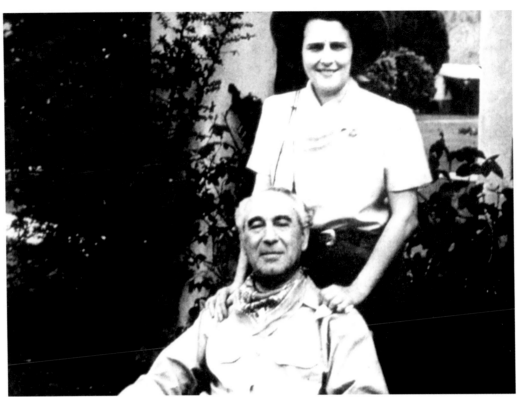

A Change in Direction

The year 1943 was hardly a great one for the Society—or for society in general. America, drawn into World War II in 1941, had troops flung across the globe. Hitler was rampaging through Europe, and the British were bombing Berlin. At home, life went on: *Oklahoma!* opened on Broadway, the Yanks thrashed the Cards in five games in the World Series, and *For Whom the Bell Tolls* was a hit at the box office.

Death went on, too. That year, one in six deaths in America was due to cancer. One of those who died was a friend of Mary Lasker's.

Lasker was charming, smart, rich, and a friend to people in the highest of places. She and her husband, Albert, were the crème of New York society, philanthropists who started a foundation in 1942 to change the way the federal government supported medical research. With money Albert had made in advertising—he named Wrigley Field, hired a struggling young comedian named Bob Hope to sell Pepsodent toothpaste on the radio, and made Sunkist a household name—the Laskers had first intended to concentrate on research into mental health and birth control. Mary Lasker became interested in cancer when a cook in her household was diagnosed with advanced uterine cancer. When the young woman's doctor said there was nothing he could do to treat the terminal disease, Lasker decided to find out what was being done to find a cure.

What she found shocked her. Almost no cancer research was under way in the United

States, save that being done by a few hospitals and privately funded scientists. Although President Roosevelt had signed the Cancer Institute Act in 1937, there was still only about seven hundred fifty thousand dollars being spent in the entire country on cancer research. The amount offended her deeply. She knew from her husband's advertising background that you needed more than that to sell tubes of toothpaste. She was equally shocked, after a conversation with the Society's managing director, Dr. Clarence Cook Little, to find that the most prominent cancer-fighting group in America did not allocate a single penny to research.

When the ASCC was founded in 1913, its primary mission was to educate the public about cancer and to encourage prompt diagnosis and treatment. Other than gathering and reporting cancer statistics, there was little interest in direct involvement with cancer research, although there had been a few nods in its direction over the years. The first effort was in 1916 when a delegation of ASCC leaders attended the International Cancer Congress in London. They met cancer research scientists from medical centers around the world whose work emphasized the importance of studying the basic nature of cancer as the key to more effective treatment and reducing cancer deaths. In 1926, the Society again took a tentative step toward sup-

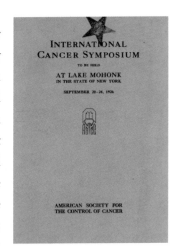

porting research when it hosted the first major international cancer conference in the United States, held at Lake Mohonk, New York. Clinicians and research scientists from major medical centers of the United States, Latin America, Europe, and Japan came to learn more about both the clinical and research aspects of cancer. Many of the research papers presented at the conference focused on laboratory attempts to identify cancer-causing agents and papers discussing the most effective treatment of malignant tumors. These included reviews of traditional surgical cancer treatment and the newer attempts to control cancer by using radium or x-ray radiation therapy.

In 1921, Elsie Mead and the New York Division of the ASCC led a campaign that successfully raised two hundred fifty thousand dollars for the purchase of a gram of radium, to be donated to Madame Marie Curie of Paris as a gift from the American people. Curie and her husband, Pierre, first isolated the element radium in 1902 and suggested it had value in the treatment of cancer. Radium was so expensive, however, the couple was unable to buy it for their own research. Several years after the first gift, the New York Division collected another two hundred fifty thousand dollars for a second gram of radium for more research.

This campaign was probably the Society's first to raise money to support a

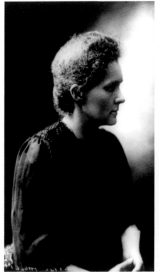
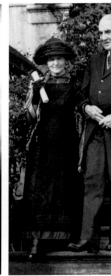

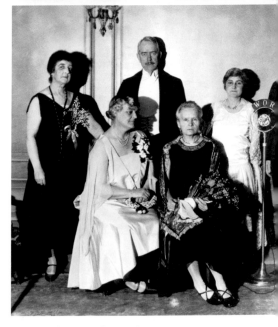

Above far left: Program for an early cancer symposium sponsored by the Society. Above top left: Marie Curie. Top right: Marie Curie and President Harding. Above: Left to right, seated: Mrs. Elsie Mead; Madame Marie Curie; standing: Mrs. Samuel Clark; Dr. Howard Canning Taylor, president of the Society; Mrs. William Brown Meloney; and Dr. John C. A. Gerster. The picture was taken prior to a dinner in honor of Curie, given in New York by the Society.

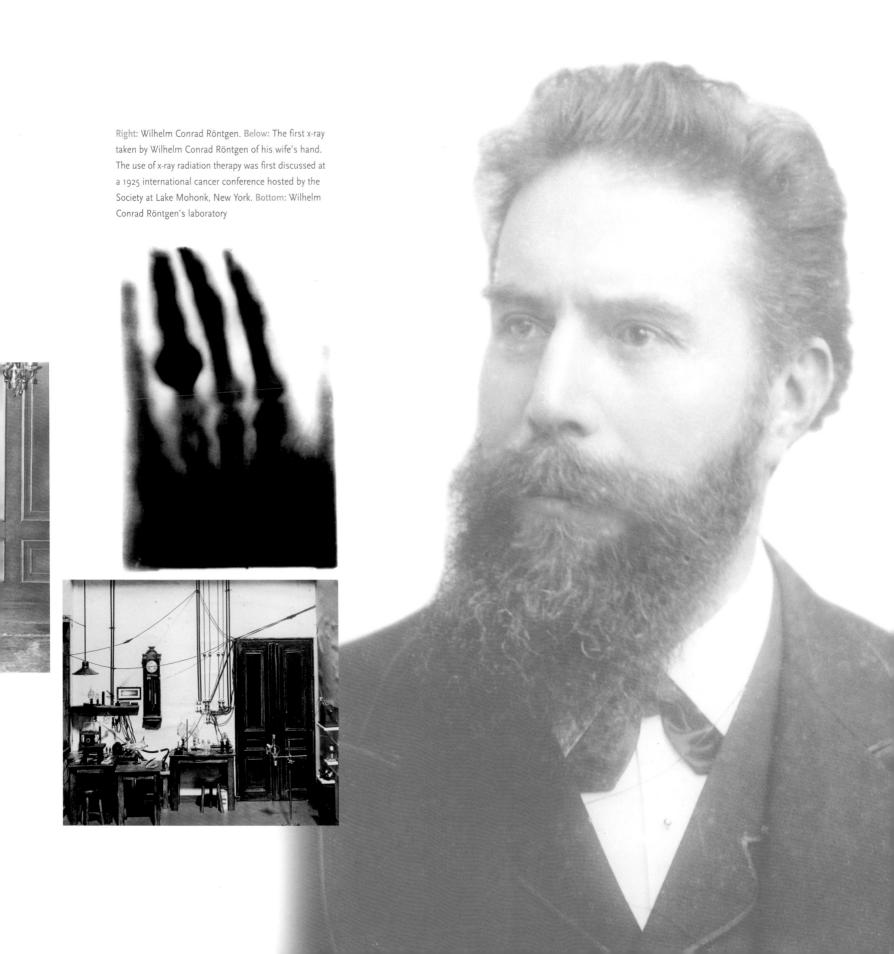

Right: Wilhelm Conrad Röntgen. Below: The first x-ray taken by Wilhelm Conrad Röntgen of his wife's hand. The use of x-ray radiation therapy was first discussed at a 1925 international cancer conference hosted by the Society at Lake Mohonk, New York. Bottom: Wilhelm Conrad Röntgen's laboratory

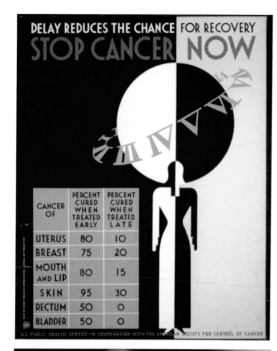

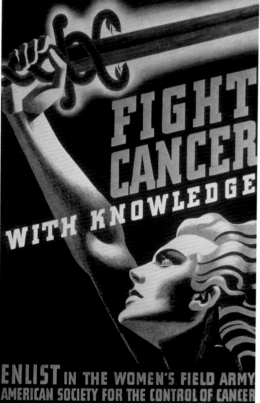

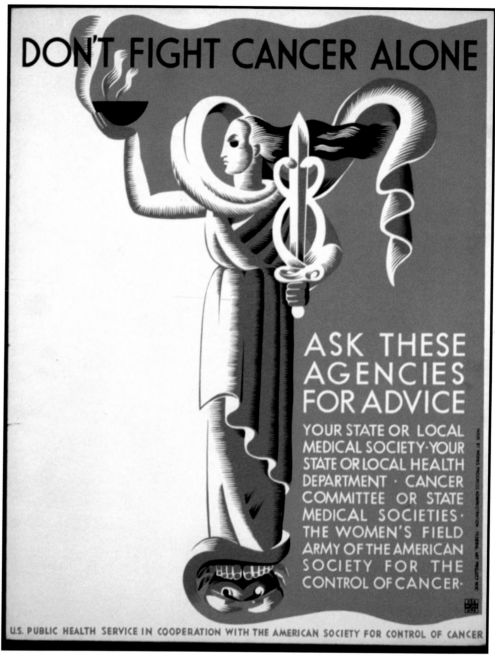

Top left and above: Posters created as part of the Works Progress Administration Federal Art Project between 1936 and 1938

Left: A recruiting poster of the Women's Field Army

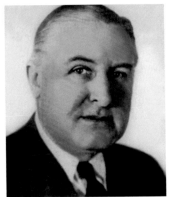

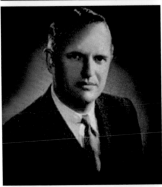

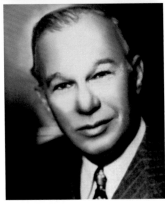

Above: Society President Dr. Frank Adair (top) was talked into "sprucing up" the Society and he, in turn, sought out advertising executive Emerson Foote (center) to do just that. Part of the plan included bringing powerful lay people onto the board, such as Elmer Bobst (bottom), a wealthy businessman.

cancer research effort directly. It was also just about its last for almost twenty years.

The leadership of the Women's Field Army had taken a small step at looking beyond education of the public for other ways to combat cancer. During the 1944 annual convention, the officers discussed the possibility of donating some money for the support of cancer research. However, that year the entire income of the ASCC was less than a million dollars from all sources. The Society's major commitment was to cancer education, and there simply were not sufficient funds to develop an effective cancer research program.

Although the National Cancer Institute Act had established the National Cancer Institute in 1937 to study the cancer problem and foster cancer research in the United States, Congress had allocated only four hundred thousand dollars. Financial aid for cancer research was extremely difficult to obtain, particularly for young researchers. Funding for cancer research was, in fact, so unpredictable and erratic that no research scientist could afford to rely solely on cancer research as a career.

None of this looked or felt right to Mary Lasker. How could you cure cancer if you weren't looking for a cure? Curious about what it would take to make an impact, she consulted with Dr. Cornelius Rhoads, a

Dr. Cornelius Rhoads

world-renowned cancer research scientist at New York Memorial Hospital, who told her that two hundred fifty thousand dollars for cancer research "given to the right laboratory would go a long way toward finding a cure for this dread disease." She talked to Dr. Frank Adair, then president of the Society, about what could happen if the ASCC was, in her words, "spruced up." She turned to her husband, Albert, whose mother had died of cancer, and convinced him to help; he, in turn, added an advertising associate, Emerson Foote, into the mix—a man who had lost both parents to cancer. Over the years, the two advertising men had developed close working relationships with executives in the broadcasting and print media—relationships that could be invaluable to the Society. The Laskers and Foote saw the possibilities: they believed, with the support of the national media, including radio broadcasting, motion pictures, magazines, and newspapers, that they could raise four million dollars in one year.

For the Society to be successful, though, the Laskers believed it needed a fundamental shift in the composition of its board and in its mission. Although the organization had lay board members from its founding, the

Society was, and had always been, controlled by physicians. Their iron grip brought respect to the ASCC but little money; the doctors weren't trained in fundraising, and the Society had for decades raised relatively small amounts of money. The Laskers and Foote believed the board needed to include some of their powerful friends, and they wanted half the board to be lay members—people like Elmer Bobst, the head of a large pharmaceutical company, known for both his philanthropy and his business and political acumen.

Then there was the question of how to spend the money. In the formula worked out years before and which still exists today, 60 percent of money raised remained in the Divisions, while 40 percent went to the National Home Office for support of nationwide programs. The Laskers wanted 25 percent—more than half of the national organization's split—to fund research. And if that weren't enough, they wanted the name of the organization changed to the American Cancer Society.

Oddly, although there were heated debates, the Laskers got what they wanted relatively easily. "Since we were only asking that research receive 25 percent of money they didn't even have yet, they must have thought, 'Well, what can we lose?' . . . So they said yes . . . and even agreed to the fifty-fifty board as well," Mary Lasker explained years later with some amusement.

And so, in 1945, the leadership of the Society agreed that to be an effective cancer

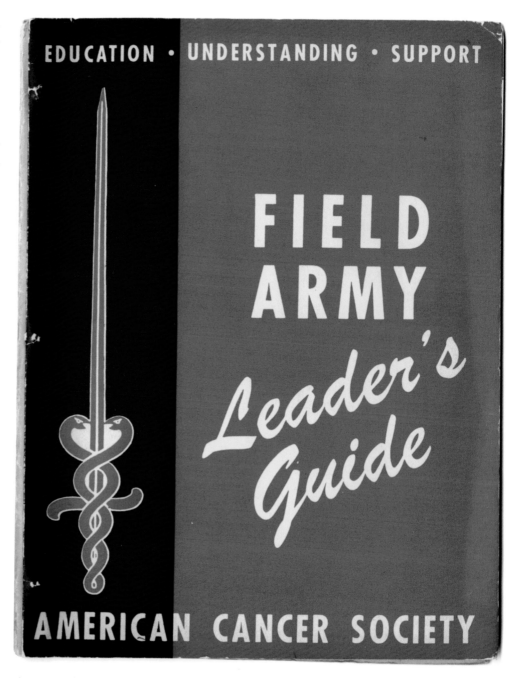

Above: In 1945, the board of directors voted to change the name of the Society to the American Cancer Society (as evidenced by this field guide), and the Women's Field Army became the Field Army of the American Cancer Society.
Opposite: 1948 cover of *Cancer News*

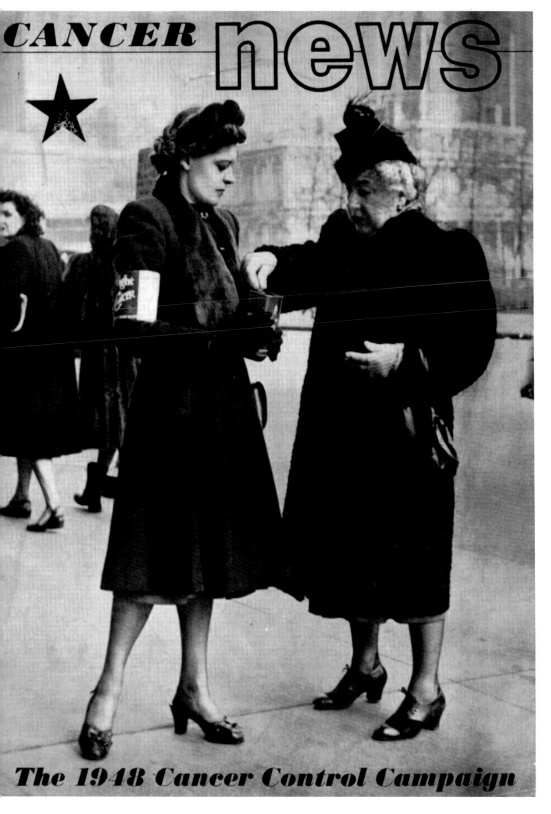

CANCER news

★

The 1948 Cancer Control Campaign

control organization, both men and women should be involved in all of its cancer-fighting activities. That year, the board of directors voted to change the name of the Society to the American Cancer Society, and the Women's Field Army became the Field Army of the American Cancer Society. At the same time, the board reaffirmed a decision made two years earlier to increase the size of the board of directors, to appoint a powerful executive committee, and for the board to be composed of equal numbers lay and medical/scientific professionals. The board also decided that the positions of president and chairman would be held by volunteers for the term of one year, and that the national president would always be a scientist or a physician, and the chairman a layperson.

The Laskers knew they could raise their money. With the help of friends in the media, they had already published a single article in *Reader's Digest*. The piece brought in one hundred twenty-nine thousand dollars—this while America was at war. The April 1945 Cancer Week, fueled by the advertising savvy of the Laskers and Foote, roared into the American consciousness with the message, "Guard those you love. Give to Conquer Cancer." So many checks came into the Society that they had to send the envelopes to a bank and have the tellers open them. Three hundred thousand dollars of that came from New Jersey, where the governor had personally asked Bobst to chair the local Division; previously, the most New Jersey had ever contributed was thirty thousand dollars. By the end of the year, the Society had four million dollars in pledges, the attention of some of the most important business leaders in America, and a new mission that included a heavy emphasis on funding research. The next year, the American public gave two and a half times more than it did in 1945, and more than ten times as much as they donated the year before that. By 1947, the national goal was twelve million dollars, and the Society met it. A Society leader, writing in 1948 about the now-named Field Army of volunteers, lauded the group as "responsible for the remarkable growth in cancer education in this country . . . The heart of the cancer control program in this country is in the ever-increasing group of . . . devoted volunteers . . . who have proved their willingness over the years to give time and money."

A Voice for Women

The success of the Women's Field Army had clearly shown the power of women as a volunteer force. Historian Jill Moffett of the University of Iowa has suggested that it was the precursor of the contemporary breast cancer movement, introducing a new way of

thinking about how to mobilize the public, particularly through women (see Chapter 4, "Doing Battle"). In many ways, it gave a voice to women—women researchers, women activists, women politicians, women political leaders—and attention to specific interests of women that were not widely known in other areas of society.

It also became the basis for the door-to-door fundraising system the Society used until the 1990s, helping create a nationwide, hands-on cancer-fighting community with untold strength across America. The "war" the Field Army was fighting was a personal, never-ending one, and the lessons learned from it—how to raise awareness and mobilize the public—are still an effective part of the Society's fundraising and information dissemination in today's highly technological and global world.

The Women's Field Army helped move women from the sidelines of the Society and ultimately altered the shape of the organization. Because of those changes, the Society rapidly grew into one of the best funded and most effective nonprofit organizations in America.

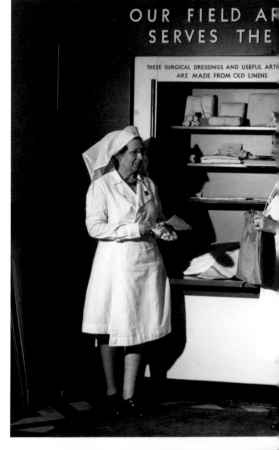

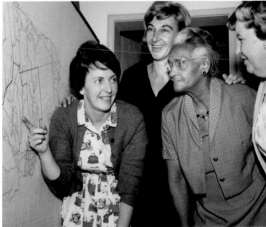

Above: Santa Cruz, California, volunteers at the start of the Society's local house-to-house fund drive, 1965. Opposite inset: Egie Huff of Georgia held virtually every volunteer position at the Society and represented the organization in its global outreach. Top: Field Army volunteers

NATIONAL WOMEN VOLUNTEER LEADERS

CHAIR, NATIONAL BOARD OF DIRECTORS

2008 — Marion E. Morra, MA, ScD
2007 — Anna Johnson-Winegar, PhD
2006 — Sally West Brooks, RN, MA
1997 — Jennie R. Cook
1988 & 1989 — Kathleen J. Horsch

NATIONAL WOMEN PRESIDENTS, AMERICAN CANCER SOCIETY

2009 — Elizabeth "Terry" T. H. Fontham, MPH, DrPH
2006 — Carolyn D. Runowicz, MD
2003 — Mary A. Simmonds, MD

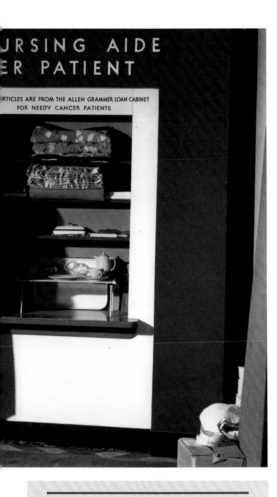

URSING AIDE
ER PATIENT

RTICLES ARE FROM THE ALLEN GRAMMER LOAN CABINET
FOR NEEDY CANCER PATIENTS

That change additionally meant missions were reshaped: women believed cancer research was as important as public information; programs were started by a woman to remind surgeons they took away more than a woman's breast when they performed a mastectomy; laws were passed because women flooded legislative offices with letters of anguish about the impact of cancer on their lives.

The Society's decision to create an organizational structure made up of men and women was not an immediate success. Men continued to dominate the national boards and committees of the organization. It was not until the late '70s and '80s that many leaders in the Divisions and Units were women. Today, about 80 percent of the volunteer force and the professional staff are women. Since the late 1980s, five national board chairs have been women.

But the work of the Field Army helped open the doors to individual women volunteers who in the last fifty years have left strong imprints on the organization: Mary Lasker used the power of her money and her intellect to change the mission of the Society at a crucial moment in its history. Helene Brown, a Medal of Honor recipient from California—"all of four-foot eleven, but a thousand-pound gorilla when it comes to fighting cancer," as a past board chair described her—pushed an agenda that made the Society more fully attendant to public health needs. Egie Huff of Georgia held

Egie Huff

almost every volunteer position at the local, divisional, and national levels and represented the Society in its global outreach. Terese Lasser drew on her strength as a breast cancer survivor to help thousands of women through the Society's Reach to Recovery® program. Kathleen "Kay" Horsch pioneered as the first woman board chair and led the Society in developing a new paradigm for community outreach. And Pat Flynn of Tacoma, Washington, helped teach the world how to put on a Relay For Life®.

Dr. John Seffrin, chief executive officer of the Society, has more than once publicly saluted the role of women in the Society. "While the Society was founded in 1913 by a small group of men, its lifeblood to grow, prosper, and spread across the nation came from the women volunteers and staff. However, for many decades the top volunteer and staff leadership positions were held largely by men."

He is also clear that era has come to a close. "More recently, through a corporate commitment and concerted follow-through efforts, many more women have come to occupy these senior-most positions of staff and volunteer leadership. While the mission of the Society will always attract a diverse group of committed people to our organization, women will, I believe, play an ever-increasing role in Society leadership positions in our destiny to eliminate cancer as a major public health problem."

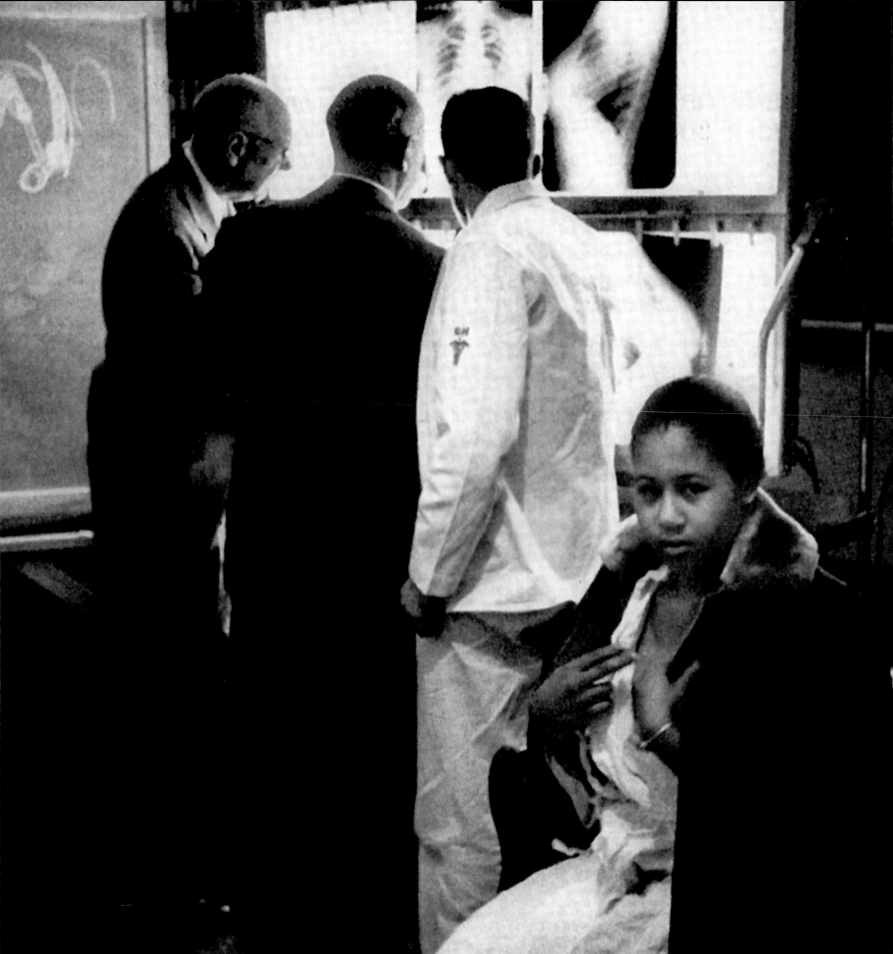

Searching for Wisdom— and Helping Pay for It

CHAPTER THREE

The 1945 change in the leadership of the organization was hugely successful for the American Cancer Society. But it was the world that profited from the addition of the research component. "Our concern was to stop all those people from dying. To stop cancer. The Society was the best weapon we had," Mary Lasker said in a 1965 interview. Of the four million dollars raised in 1945, one million was immediately allocated to research. Of the ten million dollars raised in 1946, three and a half million went to what that year's annual report called "a great nationwide coordinated program of cancer research." The structure put in place to oversee the research grants, including the organization of a rigorous peer review system and the decision to encourage young investigators to apply by funding cancer research training fellowships, has been followed for more than sixty years.

For the first half of the twentieth century, cancer had been mainly the province of surgeons. A few drugs had been tried, some derived from the mustard gas used in trench warfare in World War I. The treatments were highly toxic and mostly ineffective. However, the second half of the twentieth century promised to be an exciting time for cancer research. Between 1946 and 1952, the Society awarded more than fourteen hundred researchers grants totaling $12.2 million, institutional research grants totaling $10.3 million, and two million

Opposite: A patient in a cancer clinic, 1956

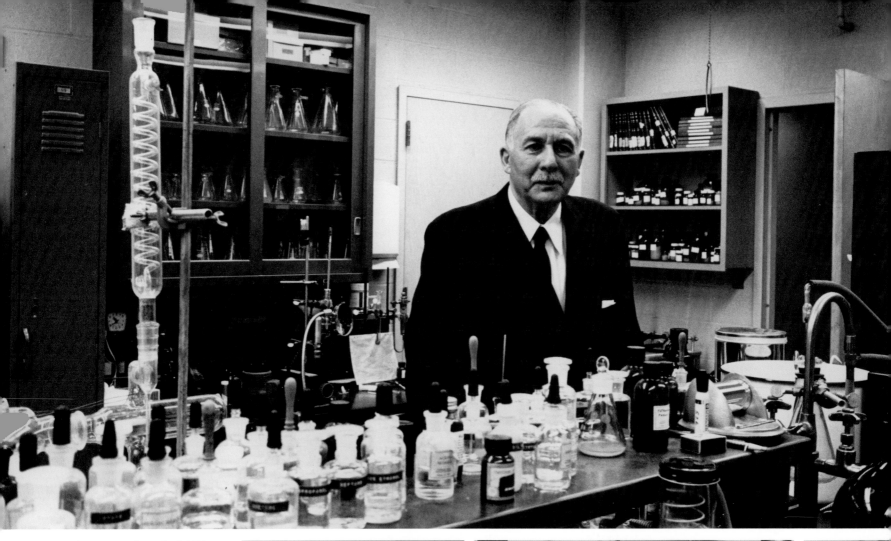

Above: In 1947, Society-funded Sidney Farber, MD, sent childhood leukemia into remission with the first successful chemotherapy. The treatment now saves thousands of lives every year. Right: This poster from the 1950s listed what were then the three main treatments for cancer. Far right: Early medical equipment may have appeared a little intimidating, but it helped immeasurably in the fight against cancer.

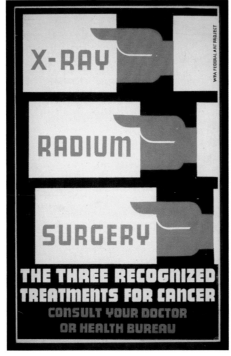

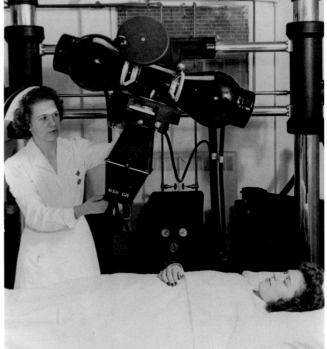

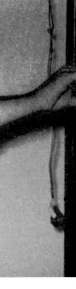

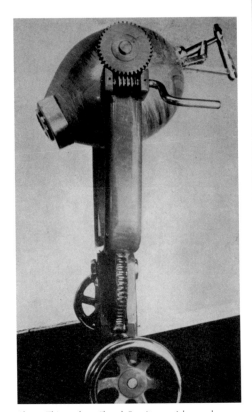

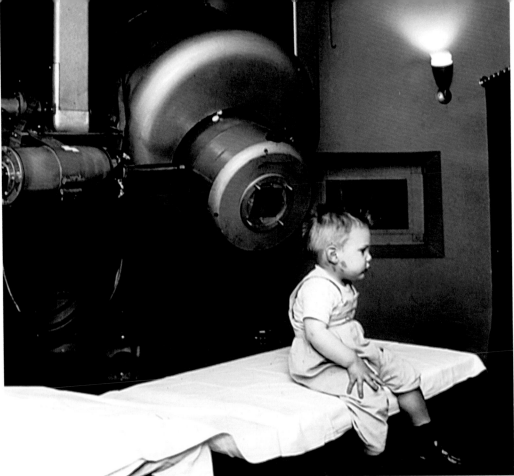

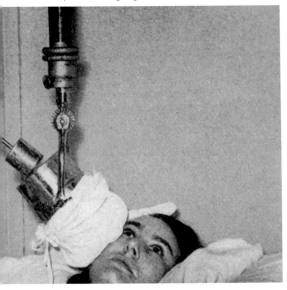

Above: This pack, or "bomb," as it was nicknamed, contained four grams of radium and was used in the treatment of deep-seated internal cancers. Right: Gordon Isaacs, the first patient treated with the linear accelerator (radiation therapy) for retinoblastoma in 1957. Below: A patient undergoing radium treatment

dollars in fellowship and scholastic grants; by 2006, the Society was awarding more than one hundred million dollars in grants annually. The early investments in research helped scientists discover cancer-causing viruses in animal tumors, with the hope that this would lead to finding the actual causes of cancer. The influence of hormones on the growth of prostate cancer and breast cancer was demonstrated and was being studied as a possible treatment. There were even reports that some types of cancer were shrinking when exposed to newly discovered chemical compounds. This development represented the beginning of the era of treatment by

chemotherapy, led by Dr. Sidney Farber, recipient of one of the Society's first research grants.

"Oncology was a new specialty that really began in the 1950s," recalls Dr. Raymond Lenhard, president of the Society in 1996 and a professor at Johns Hopkins for thirty-five years. "The [Society] recognized early that progress in research was dependent on a critical mass of physician investigators." The impact of that recognition, and the decision to provide funds particularly to what he calls the "endangered species"—young researchers—at a time when almost no one else was, was astonishing. "It became the most influential cancer research society in the world," says

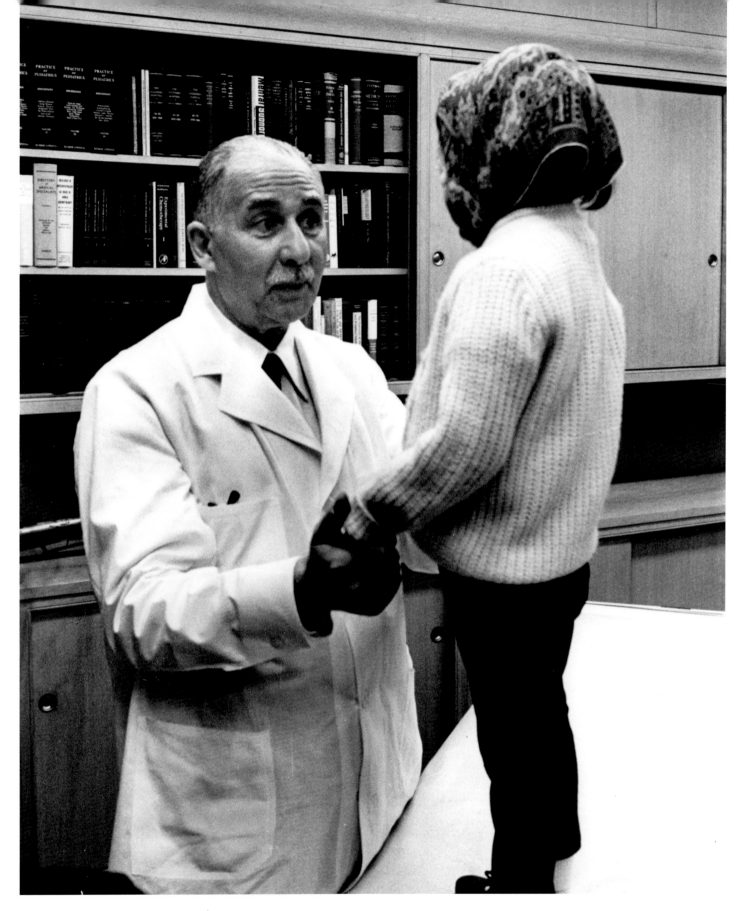

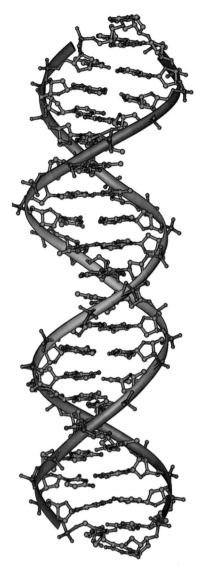

Lenhard, who himself was a Society-supported fellow while researching lymphomas and Hodgkin disease.

Over the last fifty years, the Society has helped fund some of the most groundbreaking research on cancer: Dr. Farber and his work in treating childhood

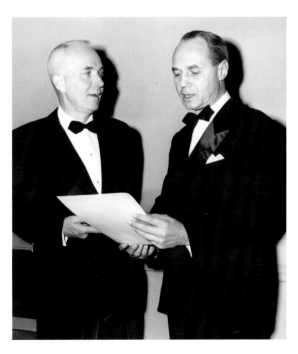

Dr. Raymond Lenhard

leukemia; Dr. Charles B. Huggins, whose Nobel Prize–winning research on prostate cancer changed forever the way scientists regarded the behavior of all cancer cells, and who, for the first time, brought hope to the prospect of treating advanced cancers; Dr. James D. Watson, whose boyhood affection for bird-watching led to a serious interest in genetics, and who, with research partner Francis Crick, discovered DNA's double-helix structure; Dr. Brian J. Druker, who discovered Gleevec, used to treat chronic myeloid leukemia, a disease that strikes approximately forty-five hundred people in the United States each year.

"The American Cancer Society has had the wisdom to support research in broad areas of basic research, some of which don't seem at first glance to affect cancer patients," says Dr. Gerald Fink, a pioneer in yeast genetics, former director of the prestigious Whitehead Institute for Biomedical Research, and a grant recipient. Pointing out that his own area of research when he was appointed an ACS research professor was "a far reach to the bedside," Dr. Fink speculated, "They must have a

crystal ball." In his case, research that began with the molecular genetics of the fungus that makes beer and bread led to a study of novel antibiotics that could relieve sometimes fatal fungal infections in cancer patients.

Ultimately, the crystal ball has allowed the Society to provide early funding to forty-four winners of the Nobel Prize. The grants also have helped attract an increasingly high caliber of affiliation with the Society itself. People like Dr. David Rosenthal and Dr. Irvin Fleming, for example—both of whom were supported by Society grants early in their careers—later became leaders in their fields and presidents of the Society.

At the same time, the Society has learned to look inside itself for some of the answers.

Opposite: Dr. Sidney Farber, shown here with a young patient, was at the forefront in the use of chemotherapy in the treatment of cancer. Above: DNA's double-helix structure was discovered by James D. Watson, PhD, and Francis Crick, MD. Top right: Dr. Raymond Lenhard was a Society-supported fellow while researching lymphomas and Hodgkin disease, and later became president of the Society. Right: Society grantee Dr. Charles B. Huggins receives the Medal of Honor from Board Member Walter Kohler, governor of Wisconsin.

BACKING WINNERS

The Society's research program has maintained a successful balance among many areas of research and supported thousands of scientists at critical times in their careers. Among those have been forty-four investigators who went on to win the Nobel Prize, a tribute to the Society's research program and the strength of its peer-review process.

| 1945 | 1946 | 1947 | 1948 | 1949 | 19 |

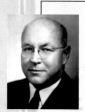

1946
Wendell Meredith Stanley, PhD (with John Howard Northrop, PhD), for the preparation of enzymes and virus proteins in a pure form

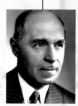

1946
Hermann Joseph Muller, PhD, for the discovery of the production of mutations by means of x-ray irradiation

| 1963 | 1964 | 1965 | 1966 | 1967 | 1968 | 1969 | 1970 | 1971 | 1972 | 1973 | 19 |

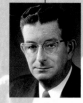

1965
Robert Burns Woodward, PhD, for his outstanding achievements in the art of organic synthesis

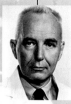

1966
Charles Brenton Huggins, PhD, for his discoveries concerning hormonal treatment of prostatic cancer

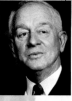

1966
Peyton Rous, MD, for his discovery of tumor-inducing viruses

1968
Robert W. Holley, PhD (with Marshall W. Nirenberg, PhD, and Har Gobind Khorana, PhD), for the interpretation of the genetic code and its function in protein synthesis

1968
Marshall Nirenberg, PhD (with Har Gobind Khorana, PhD, and Robert W. Holley, PhD), for the interpretation of the genetic code and its function in protein synthesis

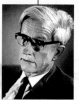

1969
Max Delbrück, PhD (with Alfred D. Hershey, PhD, and Salvador E. Luria, MD), for discoveries concerning the replication mechanism and the genetic structure of viruses

1969
Salvador E. Luria, MD, (with Max Delbrück, PhD, and Alfred D. Hershey, PhD) for discoveries concerning the replication mechanism and the genetic structure of viruses

1972
Christian B. Anfinsen, PhD, for his work on ribonuclease, especially concerning the connection between the amino acid sequence and the biologically active conformation

| 1987 | 1988 | 1989 | 1990 | 1991 | 1992 | 1993 | 1994 | 1995 | 19 |

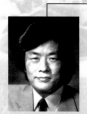

1987
Susumu Tonegawa, PhD, for his discovery of the genetic principle for generation of antibody diversity

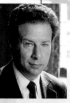

1989
Sidney Altman, PhD (with Thomas R. Cech, PhD), for the discovery of catalytic properties of RNA

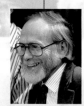

1989
J. Michael Bishop, MD (with Harold E. Varmus, MD), for the discovery of the cellular origin of retroviral oncogenes

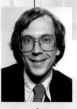

1989
Thomas R. Cech, PhD (with Sidney Altman, PhD), for the discovery of catalytic properties of RNA

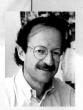

1989
Harold E. Varmus, MD (with J. Michael Bishop, MD), for the discovery of the cellular origin of retroviral oncogenes

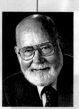

1990
E. Donnall Thomas, MD (with Joseph E. Murray, MD), for discoveries concerning organ and cell transplantation in the treatment of human disease

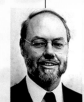

1993
Phillip A. Sharp, PhD (with Richard J. Roberts, PhD), for the discovery of split genes

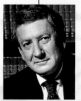

1994
Alfred G. Gilman, MD, PhD (with Martin Rodbell, PhD), for the discovery of G-proteins and the role of these proteins in signal transduction in cells

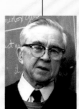

1995
Edward B. Lewis, PhD (with Christiane Nüsslein-Volhard, PhD, and Eric F. Wieschaus, PhD), for discoveries concerning the genetic control of early embryonic development

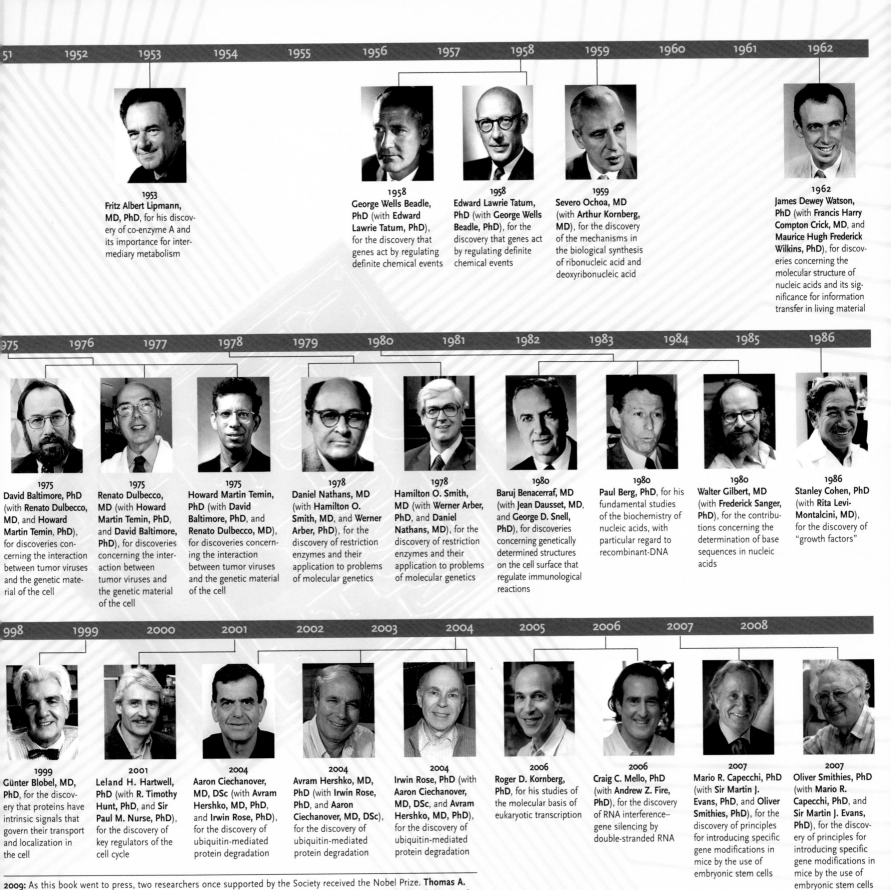

51 | 1952 | 1953 | 1954 | 1955 | 1956 | 1957 | 1958 | 1959 | 1960 | 1961 | 1962

1953
Fritz Albert Lipmann, MD, PhD, for his discovery of co-enzyme A and its importance for intermediary metabolism

1958
George Wells Beadle, PhD (with Edward Lawrie Tatum, PhD), for the discovery that genes act by regulating definite chemical events

1958
Edward Lawrie Tatum, PhD (with George Wells Beadle, PhD), for the discovery that genes act by regulating definite chemical events

1959
Severo Ochoa, MD (with Arthur Kornberg, MD), for the discovery of the mechanisms in the biological synthesis of ribonucleic acid and deoxyribonucleic acid

1962
James Dewey Watson, PhD (with Francis Harry Compton Crick, MD, and Maurice Hugh Frederick Wilkins, PhD), for discoveries concerning the molecular structure of nucleic acids and its significance for information transfer in living material

975 | 1976 | 1977 | 1978 | 1979 | 1980 | 1981 | 1982 | 1983 | 1984 | 1985 | 1986

1975
David Baltimore, PhD (with Renato Dulbecco, MD, and Howard Martin Temin, PhD), for discoveries concerning the interaction between tumor viruses and the genetic material of the cell

1975
Renato Dulbecco, MD (with Howard Martin Temin, PhD, and David Baltimore, PhD), for discoveries concerning the interaction between tumor viruses and the genetic material of the cell

1975
Howard Martin Temin, PhD (with David Baltimore, PhD, and Renato Dulbecco, MD), for discoveries concerning the interaction between tumor viruses and the genetic material of the cell

1978
Daniel Nathans, MD (with Hamilton O. Smith, MD, and Werner Arber, PhD), for the discovery of restriction enzymes and their application to problems of molecular genetics

1978
Hamilton O. Smith, MD (with Werner Arber, PhD, and Daniel Nathans, MD), for the discovery of restriction enzymes and their application to problems of molecular genetics

1980
Baruj Benacerraf, MD (with Jean Dausset, MD, and George D. Snell, PhD), for discoveries concerning genetically determined structures on the cell surface that regulate immunological reactions

1980
Paul Berg, PhD, for his fundamental studies of the biochemistry of nucleic acids, with particular regard to recombinant-DNA

1980
Walter Gilbert, MD (with Frederick Sanger, PhD), for the contributions concerning the determination of base sequences in nucleic acids

1986
Stanley Cohen, PhD (with Rita Levi-Montalcini, MD), for the discovery of "growth factors"

998 | 1999 | 2000 | 2001 | 2002 | 2003 | 2004 | 2005 | 2006 | 2007 | 2008

1999
Günter Blobel, MD, PhD, for the discovery that proteins have intrinsic signals that govern their transport and localization in the cell

2001
Leland H. Hartwell, PhD (with R. Timothy Hunt, PhD, and Sir Paul M. Nurse, PhD), for the discovery of key regulators of the cell cycle

2004
Aaron Ciechanover, MD, DSc (with Avram Hershko, MD, PhD, and Irwin Rose, PhD), for the discovery of ubiquitin-mediated protein degradation

2004
Avram Hershko, MD, PhD (with Irwin Rose, PhD, and Aaron Ciechanover, MD, DSc), for the discovery of ubiquitin-mediated protein degradation

2004
Irwin Rose, PhD (with Aaron Ciechanover, MD, DSc, and Avram Hershko, MD, PhD), for the discovery of ubiquitin-mediated protein degradation

2006
Roger D. Kornberg, PhD, for his studies of the molecular basis of eukaryotic transcription

2006
Craig C. Mello, PhD (with Andrew Z. Fire, PhD), for the discovery of RNA interference–gene silencing by double-stranded RNA

2007
Mario R. Capecchi, PhD (with Sir Martin J. Evans, PhD, and Oliver Smithies, PhD), for the discovery of principles for introducing specific gene modifications in mice by the use of embryonic stem cells

2007
Oliver Smithies, PhD (with Mario R. Capecchi, PhD, and Sir Martin J. Evans, PhD), for the discovery of principles for introducing specific gene modifications in mice by the use of embryonic stem cells

2009: As this book went to press, two researchers once supported by the Society received the Nobel Prize. **Thomas A. Steitz, PhD,** won the 2009 Nobel Prize in Chemistry for describing the ribosome and its function. He shared the award with Venkatraman Ramakrishnan, PhD, and Ada E. Yonath, PhD. **Jack Szostak, PhD,** received the 2009 Nobel Prize in Physiology or Medicine for the discovery of how chromosomes are protected by telomeres and the enzyme telomerase. He shared the award with Elizabeth Blackburn, PhD, and Carol W. Greider, PhD.

The "Crown Jewel"

The optimistic belief that a cure for cancer was just around the corner, now that dollars were flowing into research laboratories and cancer centers, gradually changed. Investigators began to realize that this complex set of diseases called cancer was affected by environment and behavior, as well as by heredity. While effective treatment and cure might be discovered through years of careful medical research, there was a growing sense that understanding the way the disease worked in the body was only one piece of the puzzle; understanding how the disease got there in the first place was equally important. For that, you needed numbers. Lots and lots of numbers.

Epidemiologic data, which Society leaders as far back as 1923 had cited as a vital part of the fight against cancer, began to take on a growing emphasis in the "new" Society. The in-house epidemiologic research department began in 1946, the same year its first extramural research grants were awarded. At the time, statistical and population-based studies of cancer were all but unknown. National cancer mortality rates, for example, had been tracked only since 1930. Those numbers already reflected a dramatic increase in cancer mortality; lung cancer deaths had risen by 500 percent between 1930 and 1946. Lung cancer was now the number one cause of cancer death in America, yet no one knew why it was showing such a precipitous surge. Without a good portrait of the various effects of cancer on the U.S. population as a whole and on specific groups in particular, the fight against cancer was, in many ways, still just guesswork.

The sea change in 1945 had introduced some turmoil into the Society. The Society had been, in the words of Elmer Bobst, "a small mom-and-pop business, content to putter along with limited results." Bobst, the Laskers, and the other new lay members on the board and executive committee were impatient to see immediate progress. Dr. Little, among others, was offended by what he felt was high-handedness and resigned after less than a year. A new position, medical and scientific director, was created. The first person appointed to that post left after a year. His assistant, Dr. Charles Cameron, filled the void.

Cameron was the son of a friend of Bobst's and was clearly a numbers man. He was the author of a statistical analysis of the frequency of cancer in the U.S. Navy, with which he served four years during World War II. He'd spent much of that time stationed at the Brooklyn Naval Hospital as chief of tumor service, and he'd already begun to realize the correlation between behavior and outcome when it came to the treatment of cancer. "In no other [disease] does the patient bear so large a share of responsibility for recognizing the subtle first signs. In no other does the patient alone influence the outcome to so great a degree," he wrote.

He (and his predecessor before him) had begun to assemble a group of scientists to

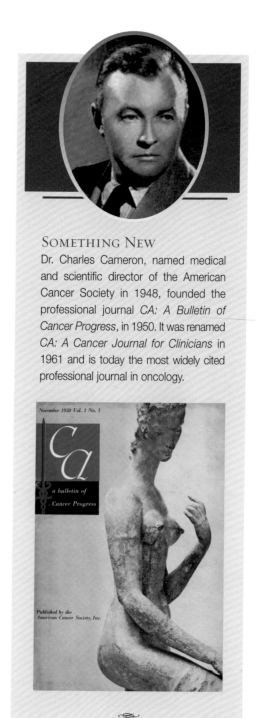

SOMETHING NEW

Dr. Charles Cameron, named medical and scientific director of the American Cancer Society in 1948, founded the professional journal *CA: A Bulletin of Cancer Progress*, in 1950. It was renamed *CA: A Cancer Journal for Clinicians* in 1961 and is today the most widely cited professional journal in oncology.

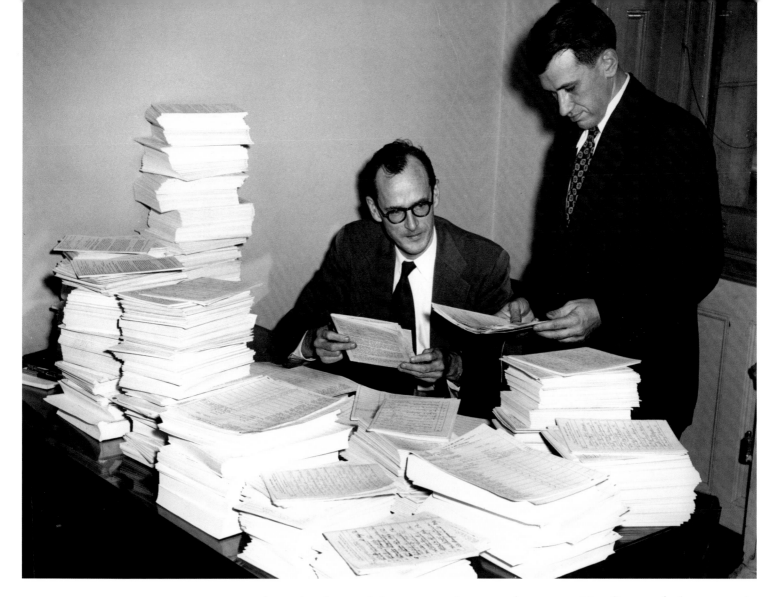

Above: Dr. E. Cuyler Hammond (seated) and Dr. Daniel E. Horn conducted a nationwide study that for the first time clearly linked tobacco usage and male lung cancer.

"In no other [disease] does the patient bear so large a share of responsibility for recognizing the subtle first signs. In no other does the patient alone influence the outcome to so great a degree,"

— Dr. Charles Cameron

gather and analyze statistics on cancer. Among those who had joined the staff was a young scientist named Dr. E. Cuyler Hammond, whose job it was to assess the effectiveness of the Society's programs and to study statistical patterns of cancer incidence and mortality. While studying at Johns Hopkins University, Hammond had first become fascinated with trends in mortality. Now the Society noticed that for nearly all forms of the disease, the mortality rates were flat or dropping—except for lung cancer. Mortality rates for lung cancer, he said, were "rising at an alarming rate."

Hammond's decision to explore why this was happening—with the backing of his boss, Cameron, and the somewhat uncomfortable approval of the board—would ultimately turn the research department into what Dr. John Lazlo calls the "crown jewel of the Cancer Society, its pride and joy." The Hammond-Horn Study, named after the two researchers, enlisted twenty-two thousand

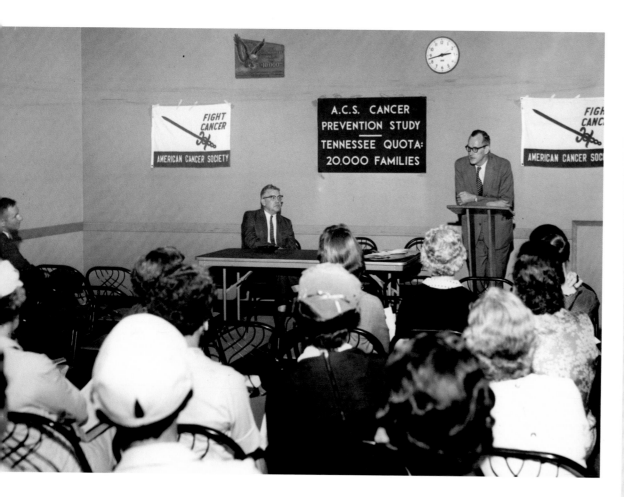

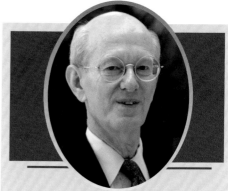

volunteers to distribute questionnaires to men nationwide. Its findings clearly linked tobacco smoking and male lung cancer (see Chapter 5, "The Tobacco Wars"). The evidence linking behavior with cancer was so strong that the Society realized it was mining statistical gold. At the same time, the melding of volunteers in helping to conduct a scientific survey was both unique and intriguing, building on and reinforcing the connection the Society was developing with communities all over the country.

In 1959, the Society launched its first Cancer Prevention Study (CPS I), which provided four hundred fifty million pieces of study information and supplied key data for the reports on smoking and health issued by the Surgeon General's office. The study provided valuable information not only on lung and other types of cancer, but on heart disease and other health issues. In 1982, its successor project, CPS II, demonstrated an increase in lung cancer among women and added to knowledge of how various medications, medical conditions, and familial and environmental factors may affect cancer risk. Cancer Prevention Study-3 (CPS-3) began

Above left: Dr. E. Cuyler Hammond speaking at a Cancer Prevention Study training session in Nashville

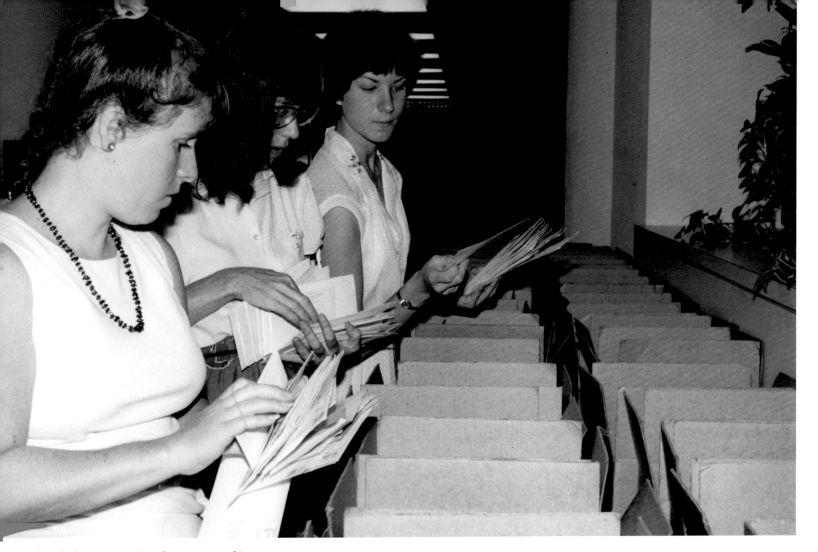

Above: Workers sort respondent information as part of Cancer Prevention Study II, 1982. Among other findings, the study demonstrated an increase in lung cancer among women. Below: As far back as 1915, coal tar was known to cause cancer, but fishermen continued to use it to coat their nets for years to follow.

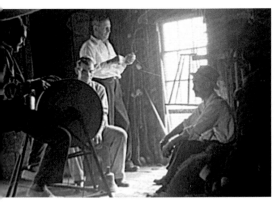

in 2007 to help scientists better understand the lifestyle, behavioral, environmental, and genetic factors that cause or prevent cancer and to ultimately eliminate cancer as a major health problem for this and future generations.

Each of these studies is used to create some of the world's largest repositories of statistical data on nonsmokers and smokers, minority populations, patients living with a diagnosis of terminal illness, patients living in poverty, and more—data that serves researchers and others seeking accurate, useful cancer information. Such data has guided almost every aspect of the Society's campaigns, from its constant battle against smoking to its decisions in the early 2000s to fight for the right for more universal access to health care (see Chapter 4, "Doing Battle").

As the body of data from the Cancer Prevention Studies grew, the Society saw other possibilities for serving the public in the fight against cancer. If, as the studies showed, people could affect their own health by the decisions they made about how they lived their lives, was there another way to help them? If people's behavior could be changed by repeated and powerful messages, could the right messages affect cancer incidence? Could people be encouraged to quit smoking? Get mammograms? And could that information also help meet the psychological and emotional needs of cancer patients?

Dr. Frederick Hoffman, a pioneer cancer epidemiologist and one of the founders of the Society, had observed more than a half century earlier that many types of cancer were the result of people's lifestyles. He also noted that delays in seeking early diagnosis and treatment were the result of human behavior patterns. Now, in the 1990s, the Society leadership began to appreciate the fact that there was much to learn about the inherent, environmental, and cultural factors that influence human behavior, particularly in people's perceptions and how they could be influenced through education. The Society was interested in funding such studies but was not receiving the kind of serious grant applications that would deserve its funding. Perhaps the best approach might be to do the research itself.

Dr. John Lazlo, a Harvard-trained researcher who had spent twenty-seven years at the Duke Medical Center teaching and doing basic research, joined the Society in 1986 as the national vice president for research. Lazlo was interested in behavioral

research but was no expert; if the Society was to become involved in this new area, he needed to know more. He decided to study one of the best cancer prevention centers in the world, in Melbourne, Australia, where a whole area of research was developing on creating effective messages about cancer. What Lazlo found was impressive. Like America, with its heavy concentration of fair-skinned European stock, Australia had seen a steadily growing problem with

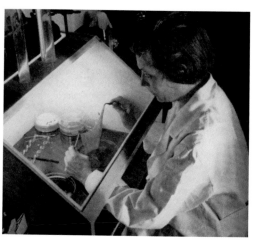

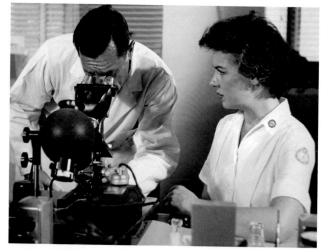

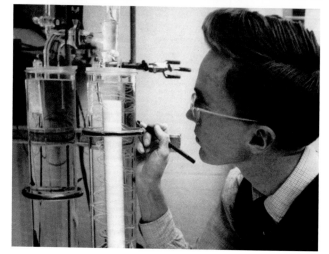

Above: A cancer researcher studies living human cells in a virus laboratory, 1956. Left: As funding began to increase, research on cancer began to grow. Bottom left: Research scientist supported by Society grants program, 1956. Opposite: Women leave the Fox California Theater after the first showings of the American Cancer Society's film on breast self-examination.

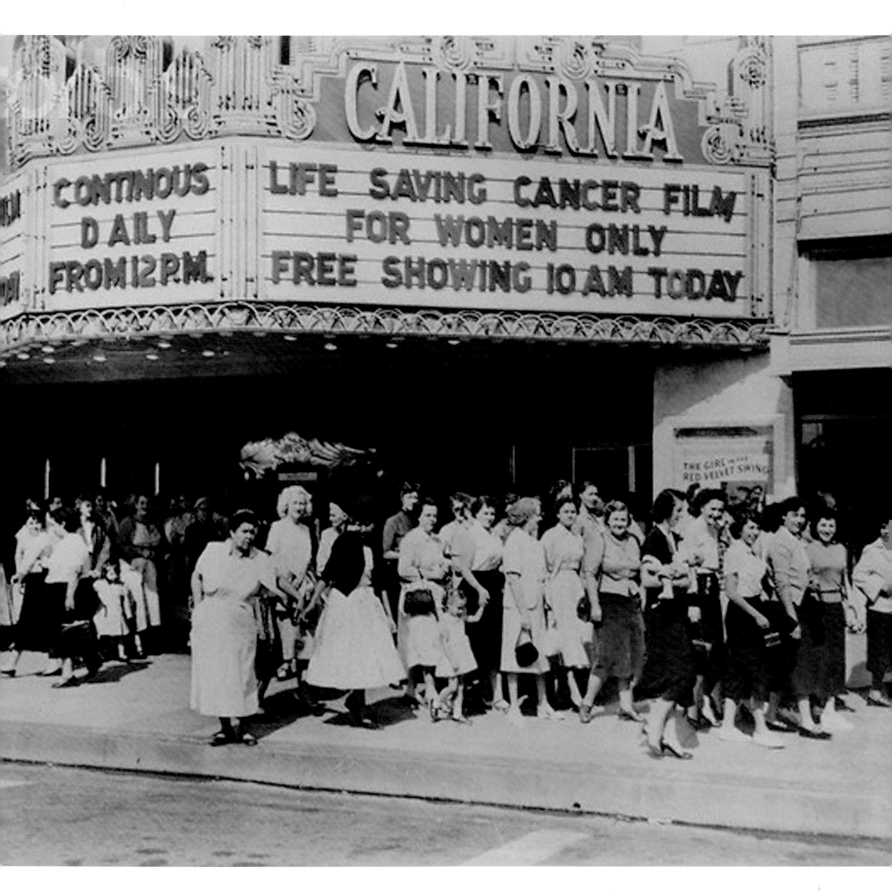

melanoma. The researchers in Australia had begun to test the kinds of messages that would convince people to protect their skin from the sun. The messages were proving extremely effective, and melanoma rates had begun to drop.

Lazlo and the Society decided that that type of research, combined with education, was adaptable to their organization, and in 1995, the Society launched its Behavioral Research Center.

Now, the Society was providing funds to outside scientists and health care professionals under a peer-reviewed grant application process that was a model for other organizations: what Dr. John Stevens, vice president for extramural grants, calls the "heart and soul of research progress, what enables us to find the best of the best." It was gathering statistical data on the causes of cancer, placing the Society squarely in a powerful intersection between the public and scientific communities. It also was producing information on building coherent messages to get people to pay more attention to early detection practices and reducing behaviors that could lead to cancer.

"Epidemiology has played a role in the American Cancer Society from the inception and made people aware of the burden of cancer," points out Dr. Harmon Eyre, the Society's former chief medical

Dr. John Lazlo

officer and executive vice president for research and cancer control science. "The first huge event was to show the link between lung cancer and tobacco."

It would hardly be the last, however.

Rethinking

There had long been a debate between those who favored targeting research grants to work on major types of cancer such as breast, prostate, lung, and colon cancer and those who wanted to support more general investigations that might still lead to significant findings. Much like the Society's earlier debates over such issues as public versus professional education, this one had both strong supporters and the potential for long-term public impact.

Public realities also guided the debate. Many things had changed since 1946, when the Society added research to its mission. At that time, the Society was the only cancer advocacy group in the United States. Almost no money was being spent on research. The U.S. government was a minor player in medicine, and "cancer politics" was not yet known. The environment had changed though, by 1995, when the Society established a blue ribbon committee, headed by Dr. Tom Burish of Vanderbilt University, to evaluate where and how it was spending its research dollars. Although the Society was

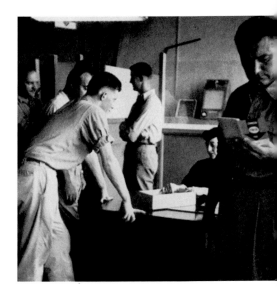

Left: After studying cancer prevention of melanoma in Australia, Dr. John Lazlo returned to America and developed a program to educate people about protection from the sun. Above: Lifesaving information can come in any form—as long as it comes. The employee education program brought cancer facts to more than three million employees of twenty-six thousand companies in 1956 by including the information in their payroll checks. Opposite: An American Cancer Society ad highlighting the Society's support of research

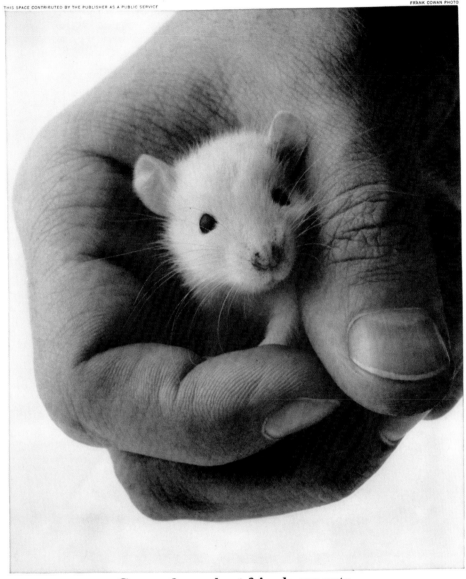

Some of your best friends are rats.

They could help save your life. They are used in research—in the laboratories of the universities and hospitals where the unceasing war against cancer is fought. Like all wars, it is expensive to wage. For instance, 1,000 rats cost $2,500—½ gram of cobalt 60 costs $6,000—one electron microscope, $35,000.

Last year, the American Cancer Society spent $12,000,000 on research to help fight this war. To cure more, give more. Every dollar helps save lives. Send your check to "Cancer," c/o Postmaster.

AMERICAN CANCER SOCIETY

distributing one hundred million dollars to research, it was a mere drop in the bucket compared to the two and a half billion dollars that the National Cancer Institute was spending on cancer research. In addition, the cancer movement had evolved into dozens of groups with special interests: women wanted more money spent on breast cancer research, leukemia and lymphoma patients wanted more attention, men with prostate cancer felt they deserved a bigger share of the research budgets.

The debate was, in some ways, a luxurious one. In days past, the question had always been simply how to find money to fund research. The American public had responded generously to the Society's message that it was fighting cancer. If that generosity were to continue—and there had been some substantial dips in giving, indicating the public needed new reassurances that its money was being used wisely—then the issue had to become how to most effectively allocate the contributions. Was it better to invest money on well-known researchers who had ongoing projects aimed at the major types of cancer, or to fund young researchers whose work might or might not lead to a major cancer breakthrough? As early as 1966, the Society's board had voted to reorganize its research program to make a focused attack on cancer through some targeted research. Now, thirty years later, the same approach was being argued.

Ultimately, the 1995 committee recommended, and the board agreed, to put the lion's share of its research money with young investigators and to set aside 10 percent of available grant money to target specific cancer problems. The first type of cancer chosen to receive the 10 percent–designated funding for cancer research was prostate cancer.

In the Hot Seat

Like so much in the Society's history, the decision was a controversial one. "We were willing to bite the bullet," says Dr. John Seffrin, chief executive officer. "Targeted research is very controversial in the research community because there's a certain tendency to say, 'Let the smart scientists decide what needs to be done.' But we also recognized that there was some research that needed to be done that, if we didn't do it, probably would never get done."

Such decisions are never easy. Just ask Dr. Michael Thun, vice president for epidemiology and surveillance research since 1988, whose own research in 1991 showed that aspirin reduced the risk of fatal colon cancer. Since then, he's gone on to become a renowned expert on the impact smoking has on the body. Whether it's defending new information linking obesity and cancer or debating the tobacco industry on numbers that show 30 percent of cancers are related to smoking, the Society is often in the hot seat—which is why, he says, it's so important to use science to affect policy decisions. Because of the strength of its in-house epidemiology center, the opinions of the American Cancer Society today are among the most highly regarded in both the public and private worlds of cancer. Thun is often called upon to give expert testimony in cancer risk–related litigation.

To date, the Society has an unblemished record of reliability, having never stated that something causes a particular cancer and then later having to retract that statement. "We believe that track record—in no small measure—is why the American people trust us and listen to what we say," says Seffrin.

The publication each year of *Cancer Facts and Figures* and the annual "Cancer Statistics" in *CA: A Cancer Journal for Clinicians*, the Society's largest-circulation medical journal, have become the most quoted publications on cancer in the world, both in mainstream and medical circles.

"Cancer Statistics," which is meant to be a reference for medical professionals, heralds the reputation of its progenitor by always starting, "The American Cancer Society estimates that . . ."

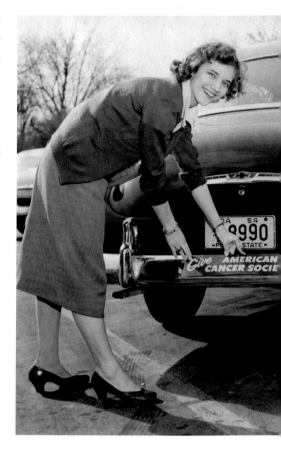

Above: Bumper sticker as part of fundraising campaign.
Left: Annually, the American Cancer Society publishes the *Cancer Facts & Figures*, a collection of statistics on cancer occurrence, deaths from cancer, and survival after diagnosis. The Society also tracks data relating to behaviors thought to influence risk and use of screening tests.
Opposite: A Society poster juxtaposed a humorous photo with a serious message—a request for funds to continue the fight against cancer.

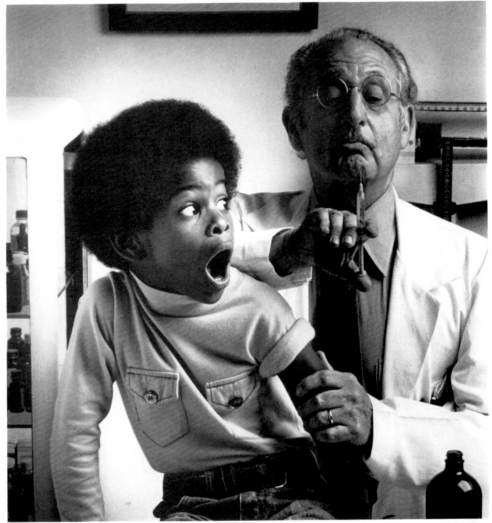

A shot against cancer?

One day the scariest thing about cancer may be the needle that makes you immune to it.

The theory: build up the body's defense to fight off a disease naturally.

Dramatic research in this direction is going on right now.

Scientists are working on mechanisms to make the body reject cancer.

And the promise for the future is staggering.

Wouldn't you feel good knowing you contributed to the research?

Feel good.

Please contribute. Your dollars will help further *all* our cancer research.

We want to wipe out cancer in your lifetime.

American Cancer Society

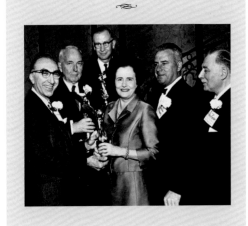

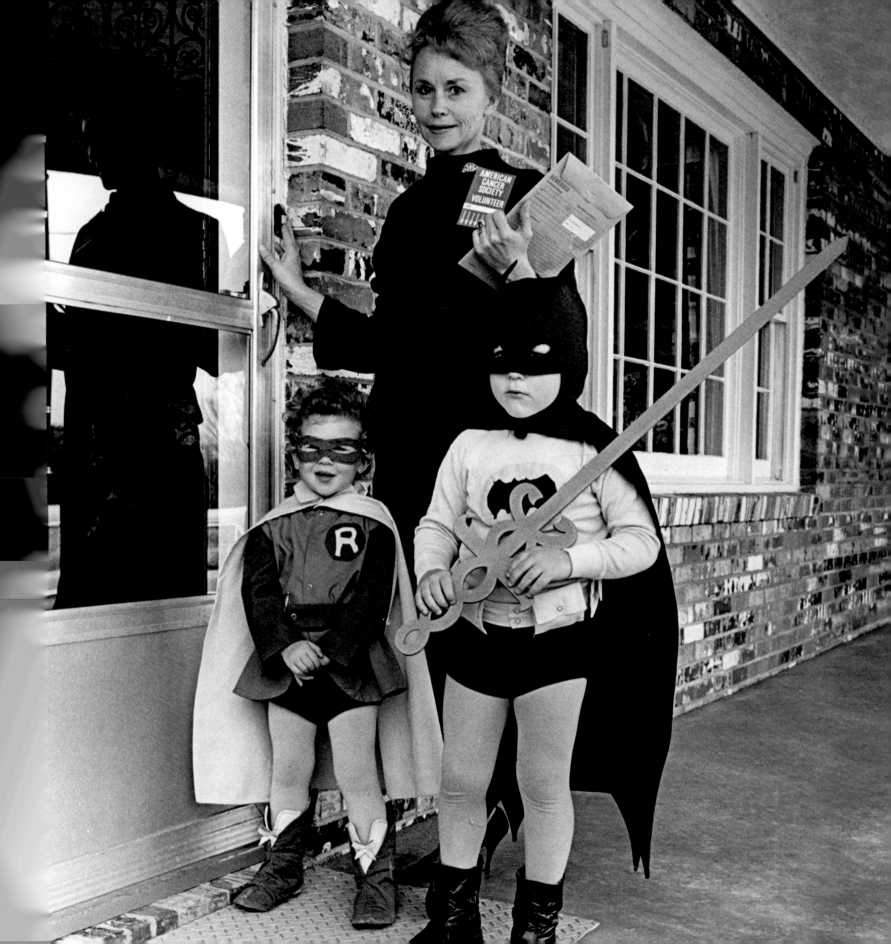

Doing Battle:
Crusades and Campaigns

Opposite: Mrs. Howard Goldman and her children in Chesapeake, Virginia, conducting a residential solicitation

Margaret Mead is quoted as saying, "We are continually faced with great opportunities which are brilliantly disguised as unsolvable problems." Here are the problems:

- More than 1.4 million new cancer cases and 562,340 deaths from cancer are expected in the United States in 2009.
- When deaths are aggregated by age, cancer has surpassed heart disease as the leading cause of death since 1999 for those younger than age eighty-five.
- African American men and women have 36 percent and 17 percent higher death rates from all cancers combined than white men and women, respectively.
- Compared with whites, other ethnic groups have higher rates for stomach, liver, and cervical cancers. Furthermore, minority populations are more likely than white populations to receive a diagnosis of advanced-stage cancer.

Here are the opportunities:

- For women, the death rate from all cancers combined decreased by 0.8 percent per year from 1994 to 2002 and 1.6 percent per year from 2002 to 2005. For men, it decreased by 1.5 percent from 1993 to 2001 and 2 percent per year from 2001 to 2005.
- Progress in reducing the burden of suffering and death from cancer can be accelerated by applying existing cancer control knowledge across all segments of the population.

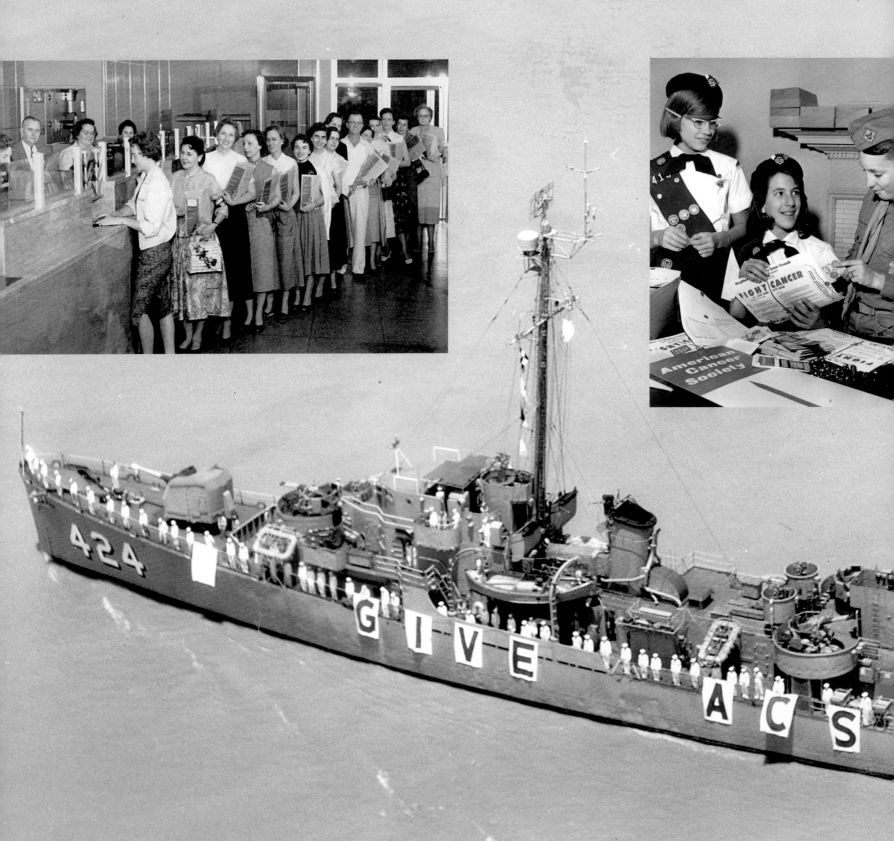

The American Cancer Society

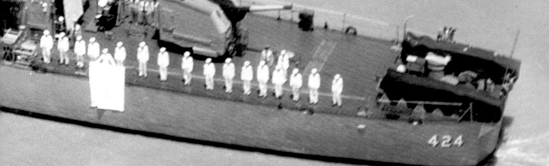

Background photo: The Destroyer Escort, USS *Haas*, steams out to join her sister ships in a dramatic anticancer maneuver of the Eighth Naval District on the Mississippi River to call attention to the 1955 Cancer Crusade. Opposite far left: After raising money, Society volunteers "stop by the bank" to make a deposit. Opposite left: Scouts stuff envelopes in support of the 1967 Cancer Crusade, working after school in the office of the Denver Unit, Colorado Division.

That last "great opportunity" has been of interest to the leaders, volunteers, and staff of the American Cancer Society for nearly one hundred years.

The Society from its genesis viewed its mission as a battle against an insidious enemy that knew no boundaries and could sneak into any community. The first "crusade"—a word chosen for its gladiatorial fierceness—was simply to remove the sense of shame, secrecy, and hopelessness the word "cancer" generated. The campaigns that followed were fed by the Society's stubborn refusal to accept that cancer can bring only death.

The Society had conducted Cancer Weeks since the early 1920s, officially labeling these national fundraising and information-sharing efforts "crusades" when the Women's Field Army in the 1930s became the militant symbol of the Society's work. Its influence was so great that in the 1930s and 1940s you could simply write the word "cancer" on an envelope for a donation, and it would be sent to the American Cancer Society. The crusades would eventually become the basis for the Unit system, in which volunteers went house to house in their communities, handing out cancer materials and collecting donations

from their neighbors. The Unit system drew in vast numbers of volunteers. Eventually, the word "crusade" would be supplanted by less warlike terms—activities, campaigns, efforts—that nevertheless captured the spirit of the great fight being waged against cancer, person by person, diagnosis by diagnosis, as cancer-prevention programs grew in scope and sophistication. By the early 1950s, the Society embarked on what would be the defining campaign in the modern cancer-fighting effort, one that would remake not only the Society but also the history of the world, when it tackled the link between tobacco use and cancer (see Chapter 5, "The Tobacco Wars").

The Society has gone on to bring its penetrating power to the fight against breast cancer, colorectal cancer, prostate cancer, and the racial and economic disparities in cancer treatment. The Society has added to the understanding of contributing health issues like obesity, nutrition, and environmental carcinogens, and it has made quality of life for cancer patients an ongoing campaign (see Chapter 8, "The Warm Hand of Service"). Within the last few years, it has begun a major campaign for a more collaborative approach to integrated health care and access to health care for all, what people inside the Society are referring to as "the twenty-first century crusade" (see Chapter 10, "2015 and Beyond").

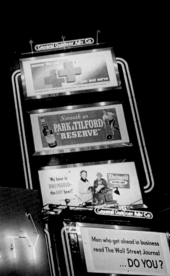

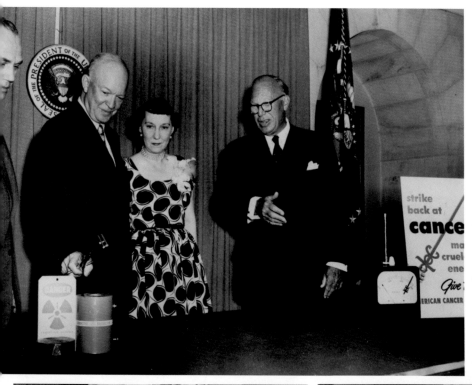

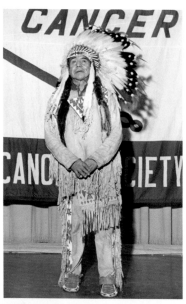

Opposite and far left: President Dwight D. Eisenhower opened the 1954 fundraising and educational crusade by lighting from Washington, D.C., a seventy-foot Sword of Hope—the symbol of the Society—in Times Square in New York City. The president used radioactive cobalt—cobalt 60—in lighting the sword. As the president brought the cobalt 60 source within range of a Geiger Counter, the amplified sound of clicks—recording radiation—were heard, building up to the final impulse that was transmitted by wire to Times Square, thus turning on the lights on the sword. Left: Alex Tohet, talent show benefit for the Society, 1962. Bottom left: Mrs. Robert Ringle, Los Angeles County residential chairman, 1965 Cancer Crusade. Bottom: A young supporter sells plaques to raise money for the Society.

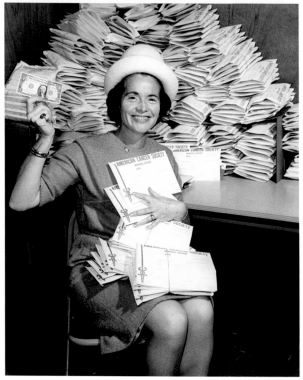

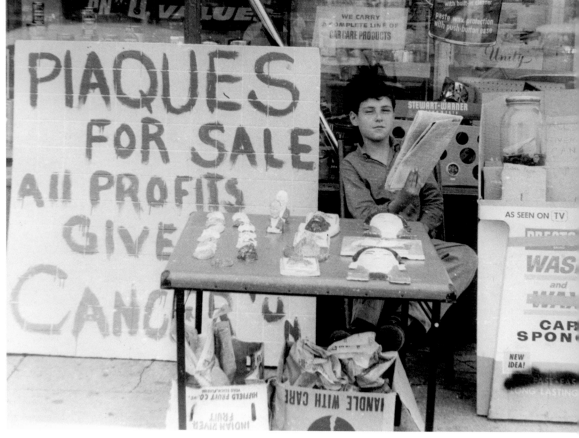

However, the first successful precursor of all these campaigns—and, along with the antismoking movement, the primitive model for later informational and advocacy efforts—would get its start in the 1940s. It began with the research of a quiet, gentlemanly scientist working six or seven days a week in an unairconditioned office that, because of fate or luck or just plain great opportunity, was across the street from where Dr. Charles Cameron, the new director of the Society and a member of the surgical staff at Memorial Hospital, did his own work.

Dr. George Papanicolaou emigrated from Greece with his wife, Mary, in May 1913, the same year and month the Society was established. When he met Cameron, he had been at Cornell University Medical Center in New York City as a research biologist for almost thirty-five years. Years earlier, while doing unrelated research, Papanicolaou discovered that cancer of the cervix could be diagnosed before it was visually evident by a fairly simple test involving vaginal cell smears. He published his findings in 1928 in a short paper that created little interest in the scientific and medical community, except to earn him the label of a "storyteller" whose work had no positive application.

Death from cervical cancer was a mind-numbing sure bet. There were no specific symptoms for early diagnosis. It seemed to develop abruptly and usually advanced to a serious condition in a few months. It meant almost certain death: in 1940, it was killing

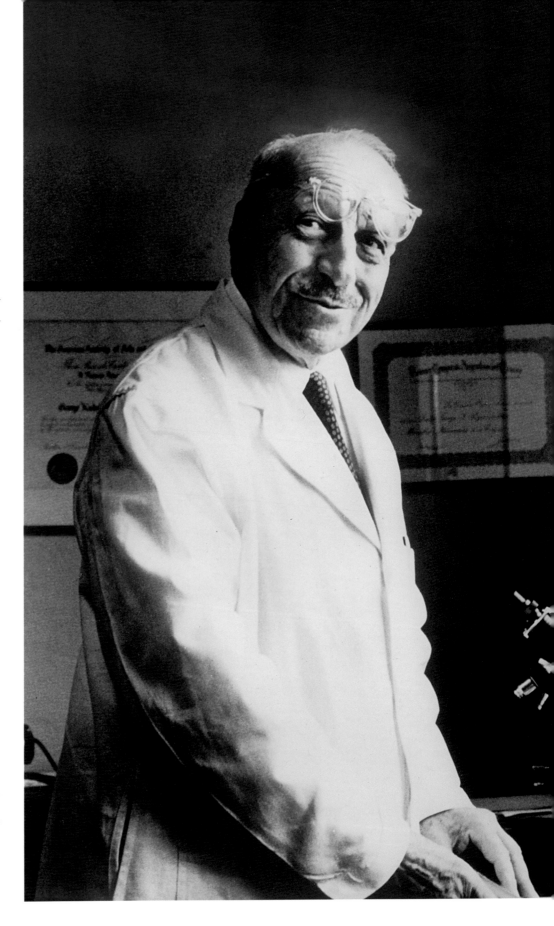

The American Cancer Society

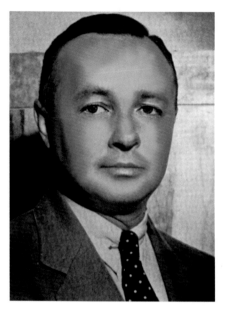

Above: Dr. Charles Cameron, a medical and scientific director of the Society, used statistics when waging his battle against cancer. Left: An immigrant from Greece, Dr. George Papanicolaou discovered in 1928—to little notice—that cancer of the cervix could be detected before it visually appeared by using a simple vaginal cell smear. It wasn't until women began to demand the test that the Pap smear became widespread. Right: It fell to Dr. Arthur Holleb, recently discharged from the navy, to try to spread the word about the viability of what became known as the Pap smear.

thirty women per one hundred thousand each year. When medical students from Cornell, across the street from Memorial, began telling Dr. Cameron about what he later described as "this guy who had discovered a test for early cancer of the uterus," Cameron, named the director of the Society in 1948, decided to walk across the street to meet him.

Cameron was intrigued. After consulting with some of the leading cancer researchers in the country, he became convinced that cytology, the study of cell anatomy, "could find cancers even where the surgeon couldn't see them." Cameron believed he was seeing a great opportunity to save lives, a crusade worth launching.

Now, all he had to do was convince the rest of the world.

A Traveling Salesman

Cameron began by pushing the American Cancer Society to what he called "full tilt." He hired a recently discharged navy lieutenant, Dr. Arthur Holleb, to take the show on the road. While in the military, Holleb had treated cancer patients at the Brooklyn Navy Hospital under Dr. Cameron, who had been chief of tumor services there. Now, Cameron asked Holleb to become a traveling salesman for the new "Pap test," making appointments with leading gynecologists and pathologists at medical centers around the country and visiting the Divisions and Units of the Society to tell volunteers about it. Holleb, who later became the Society's senior

vice president for medical affairs, spent nine months hopping trains and planes, pushing the new test, getting thrown out of offices, and convincing practically no one that this new test was worth using.

Cameron planned a National Cytology Conference in Boston in 1948. The conference met with limited success, though in later years, national conferences such as these were to become a pattern for the Society, bringing together national and international experts to address important cancer issues. The Society mainly heard the doctors' objections, which boiled down to two questions: why the test was an improvement over current methods, and who would be responsible for reading the smears.

Again, Cameron pushed the Society to provide the answers, designating money in 1950 for fifteen laboratories to properly train technicians. Using contacts made through the

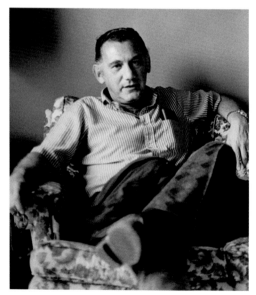

Dr. Arthur Holleb

Board, he had films produced for both lay people and physicians to explain the new test. Progress, however, was slow—and would remain so until women themselves began to demand the test. "It was the power of American womanhood that ultimately sold the Papanicolaou smear," Holleb asserted years later.

One of those women was Helene Brown, a twenty-year-old student at the University of California Los Angeles, who became a lifelong supporter and volunteer for the Society after a trip to her doctor's office in 1950 to get a pregnancy test for her first child. When her doctor, one of a few progressive gynecologists who had begun to use the test, mentioned the Pap smear, she was dumbfounded. If this was a lifesaving test, then why wasn't it being given to all women? And why had she never even heard about it? Her questions eventually led her to the American Cancer Society.

She already knew what cancer could do. As a sixteen-year-old, she had given nightly morphine shots to her father while he was dying of lymphoma. She had moved on to have two children, help her husband build his boat dealership, and complete her education as a business administration major. It was a practical degree, one that would guarantee

Helene Brown

her a job. But the impractical side of her led to a minor in biology that fed her interest in the sciences. That interest led Brown to become an advocate for public health and the issues raised by the Society for more than fifty years.

She helped bring the film Cameron had developed about the Pap smear to large theatres and Rotary and women's groups in the Los Angeles area, dragging a sixteen-millimeter projector and movie anywhere people would

EMPTY PROMISES: DEBUNKING THE MYTHS

There have always been questionable cancer remedies that promise magical cures, though often at enormous monetary and emotional expense to cancer patients and their families. For years, the Society maintained one of the most extensive collections of information and facts on unproven or alternative methods of cancer management. In the 1970s, the Society began working actively to educate the public and medical community on the facts and possible dangers of these methods.

In 1976, a national Cancer Quackery Workshop mapped a broad plan to disseminate information on unproven methods. Helene Brown, a volunteer and public health leader from California, maintained a veritable museum in her home for years, including material from conventional-looking drugs to bizarre compresses, diet machines, and other things promising to save cancer patients from the things they feared most: pain, disfigurement, expense, uncertainty, and death. As part of her research, Brown made more than one trip incognito to cancer "clinics" in Mexico, posing as a cancer patient.

Despite the years spent trying to convince the public to avoid such efforts, people are often still lured into these types of treatments, spurred by desperation and hope. Sadly, many treatments rob patients of precious months or even peaceful deaths, as well as squandering funds and delaying proven treatment that could mean the difference between life and death.

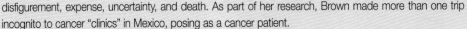

Left: Dragging a projector and screen anywhere she was allowed, Helene Brown showed a film about the Pap smear. Soon, women all over the country were doing the same. Opposite: Dr. George Papanicolaou examining a slide

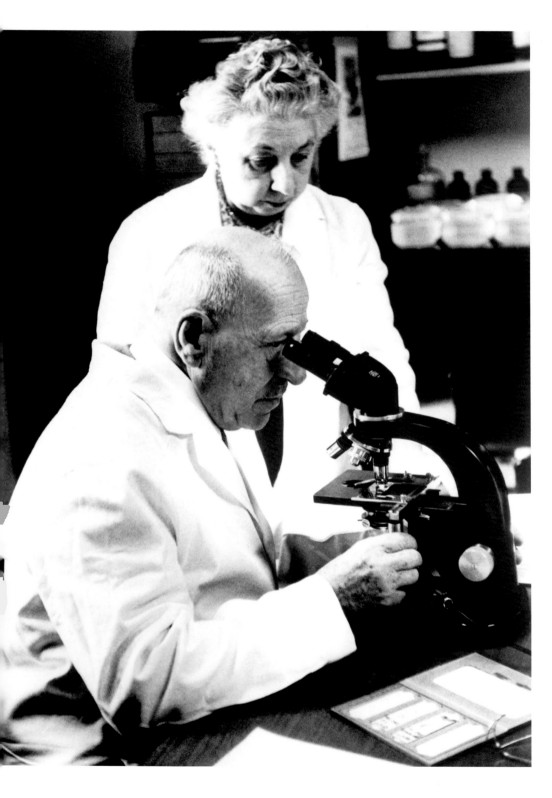

let her. "I saw firsthand what you could do by talking. I also saw that the Society did one fantastic job in selling the Pap test," she says.

All over the country, other men and women began talking and dragging projectors around, promoting the Pap campaign. In 1951, Cameron proposed to the Society's Medical and Scientific Committee, the powerful group that governed nearly all Society decisions, that they support a program to study the effectiveness of the vaginal smear in population screenings. A year later, a large, five-year study using the Pap smear was begun in Memphis, Tennessee. The study was sponsored by the Public Health Service, the University of Tennessee, the Memphis Unit of the American Cancer Society, and community physicians. Dr. Papanicolaou spent a number of months in Memphis overseeing the project, which was accompanied by an extensive advertising and promotional program—even getting a former Miss America, who was from Memphis, to promote it.

The Memphis Project proved that mass screenings were practical, and that the routine use of the Pap smear in asymptomatic women would save lives through early diagnosis. In the intervening fifty-odd years, cervical cancer has moved from the second-leading cause of cancer death in women to the thirteenth, with 4,070 deaths estimated in 2009—down from the 35,000 who died annually before the screening's acceptance as an important part of gynecologic care.

A Brilliant Attack

Promoting the Pap smear was something entirely new, the first successful cancer-prevention program ever. The widespread mass application of the Pap test was achieved faster and probably better than any new discovery, and its success emboldened and refined the Society's efforts to reach both the public and the professional community.

What the Society had discovered was a sophisticated addition to its arsenal, which now enabled a three-pronged approach: research, education, and service. It would become what Allan K. Jones, a pioneer industrial developer in the Los Angeles area who became chairman of the Society in 1981, described as "a brilliant attack."

Following the Pap smear efforts, and dovetailing with the tremendous impact of the Hammond-Horn Report about smoking (see Chapter 5, "The Tobacco Wars"), the Society began to launch efforts focusing on major types of cancer—where prevention or early detection could save the greatest number of lives—and to look at issues contributing to both the disease and its mortality rate.

Breast cancer has for decades in the United States been the leading cancer among women and the second leading cause of cancer death in women. The disease attacks the breast more often than it does any other organ. A lump in the breast, detected by self-examination, was one of the first of the famous seven warning signs of cancer the Society regularly included in its early literature. The

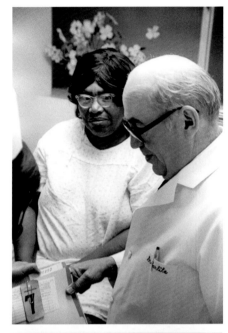

graphics used at that time by the Society were filled with very unsubtle imagery to encourage women to go to their doctors if they had a suspicious lump: if you did not go, your fate was shown as a gravestone; if you did, it was shown as a healthy body.

Unfortunately, finding a lump was difficult and meant the tumor was already late-stage. In the 1970s, in an effort to improve early diagnosis rates, the Society began a project called the Breast Cancer Detection Demonstration Project (BCDDP), in collaboration with the National Cancer Institute. The test was centered on mammography, a low-dose x-ray of the breast that had been around for years, though the quality of the imagery was initially very poor. It was not until the 1960s and '70s, with efforts led by five physicians (all past or future Society presidents), that research showed the reliability of mammography to find even smaller cancers—often smaller than one centimeter in diameter. Like surgeons in earlier eras, when radical mastectomies were the only hope for women with breast cancer, radiologists in this era became what Dr. Barron H. Lerner, an associate professor of medicine and public health at Columbia University, calls the "saviors" of women for their use of mammography to find these small and curable cancers.

Yet the BCDDP was not without controversy. The project provoked a firestorm in the mid-1970s from a few scientists who claimed that the hazards of x-ray exposure in women under fifty would outweigh any

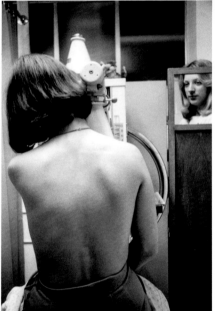

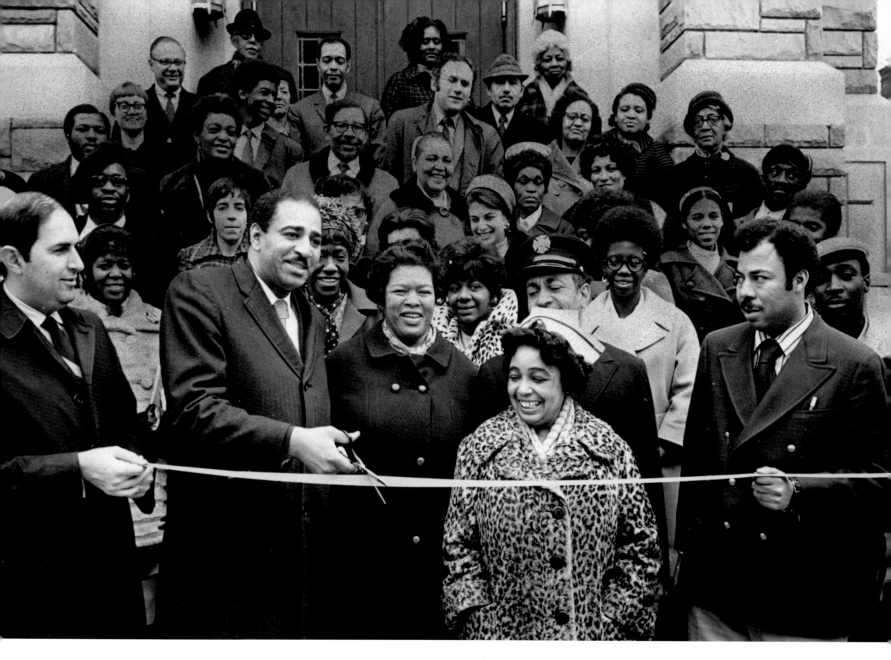

Opposite top: A patient with Dr. Thomas Carlile, who headed the Breast Cancer Detection Demonstration Project at Virginia Mason Medical Center. Opposite bottom: Woman getting a mammogram as part of the Breast Cancer Detection Demonstration Project. Above: A three-day Health Fair in Bedford-Stuyvesant, one of Brooklyn, New York's most densely populated communities. The fair was organized by thirty-five health agencies, including the Brooklyn Unit of the New York Division of the American Cancer Society. Two of the seven free clinics were offering Pap tests and breast examinations.

benefits. Explosive headlines created a "mammography war" in which the Society was accused of letting its zeal to cure cancer get in the way of its science. Opponents claimed that the mammograms themselves were so flawed that they were leading to erroneous diagnoses and unnecessary mastectomies. The fight was bitter and lasted for years. It

began to recede in 1984 when Dr. Gerald D. Dodd, then a resident at the University of Cincinnati Hospital in Ohio, issued a report saying, "It is reasonable to conclude that the potential benefits of mammography far outweigh the minimal risk incurred by the examination." Dodd was later to become president of the Society in 1991.

"YES, THERE IS LIFE AFTER BREAST CANCER. AND THAT'S THE WHOLE POINT."

—Ann Jillian

A lot of women are so afraid of breast cancer they don't want to hear about it.

And that's what frightens me.

Because those women won't practice breast self-examination regularly.

Those women, particularly those over 35, won't ask their doctor about a mammogram.

Yet that's what's required for breast cancer to be detected early. When the cure rate is 90%. And when there's a good chance it won't involve the loss of a breast.

But no matter what it involves, take it from someone who's been through it all.

Life is just too wonderful to give up on. And, as I found out, you don't have to give up on any of it. Not work, not play, not even romance.

Oh, there is one thing, though. You do have to give up being afraid to take care of yourself.

✝AMERICAN CANCER SOCIETY®
Get a checkup. Life is worth it.

Created as a public service by Ally Gargano/MCA Advertising LTD.

Twenty-five years after the study began, Dr. Myles Cunningham, president of the Society in 1997 and a surgical oncologist at St. Francis Hospital in Evanston, Illinois, wrote in an editorial in the journal *CA*, "It [BCDDP] stimulated relentless and effective efforts" to improve the overall standards of mammography performance—which allowed the BCDDP to "ultimately be judged to be one of the epochal detection trials of the last half century."

Using what it had learned from the BCDDP and other research, the Society in 1986 launched a major campaign promoting breast cancer detection, with an emphasis on the benefits of mammography. The campaign was comprehensive and interdepartmental, involving professional and public education, and became the theme of the 1987 Cancer Crusade. It used the most sophisticated public outreach tools of the day, including an endorsement from a blond bombshell: Ann Jillian, elevated to sex-symbol status by a television series, who became a Society spokesperson after she was diagnosed with breast cancer, telling women in a national ad campaign, "Yes, there is life after breast cancer. And that's the whole point."

∝

The campaign received unexpected attention when First Lady Nancy Reagan was diagnosed with breast cancer in late 1987 after a mammogram detected a cancer seven millimeters in diameter in her left breast.

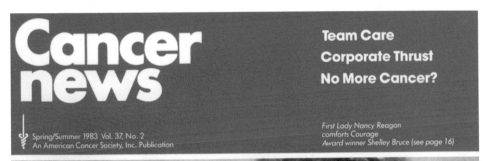

Cancer news

Spring/Summer 1983 Vol. 37, No. 2
An American Cancer Society, Inc. Publication

Team Care
Corporate Thrust
No More Cancer?

First Lady Nancy Reagan
comforts Courage
Award winner Shelley Bruce (see page 16)

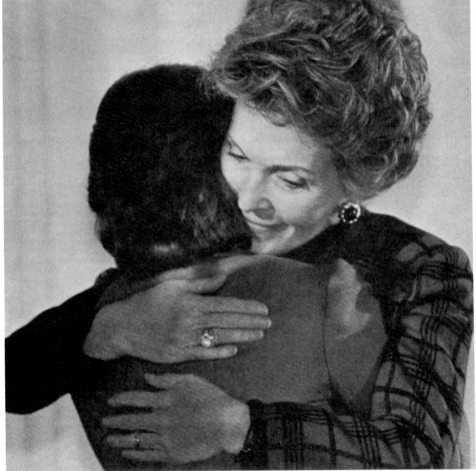

Opposite: The Society didn't hesitate to tap celebrities when promoting their message, as they did when using Ann Jillian. Above: After Nancy Reagan publicized her own mastectomy in 1987, there was a 12 percent increase in women seeking mammograms.

Mrs. Reagan didn't have the luxury of privacy, so she did the next best thing: she drafted her diagnosis and subsequent mastectomy into a kind of national teachable moment. That year, the U.S. Centers for Disease Control recorded a 12 percent increase in women seeking mammograms. They speculated the jump was the result of both Mrs. Reagan and the media attention being paid to cancer control promotions that year. (A little over a decade earlier, in 1974, both the president's and vice president's wives, Betty Ford and Happy Rockefeller, were diagnosed with breast cancer, before mammography was an accepted diagnostic tool, and underwent radical mastectomies.)

Disparities and Inequities

Continually searching for ways to teach people how to improve their own health, the Society began a nutritional focus in 1989 to reinforce the potential for cancer risk reduction. Building on that, researcher Dr. Eugenia Calle, managing director of analytic epidemiology, reported in 2003 that ninety thousand cancer deaths could be prevented each year if Americans could just maintain a normal, healthy body weight. The information emerged from CPS II, which began in 1982 and is following more than 1.2 million men and women to determine the role of environmental and lifestyle factors in cancer deaths.

By now, the Society had reported on what happened to smokers. They'd looked at some environmental and workplace carcinogens like asbestos. They knew the outcome for women who didn't get mammograms. And, in the mid-1980s, they began to examine another grim reality of American society: a huge percentage of overweight, smoking Americans with poor nutrition and inadequate health care

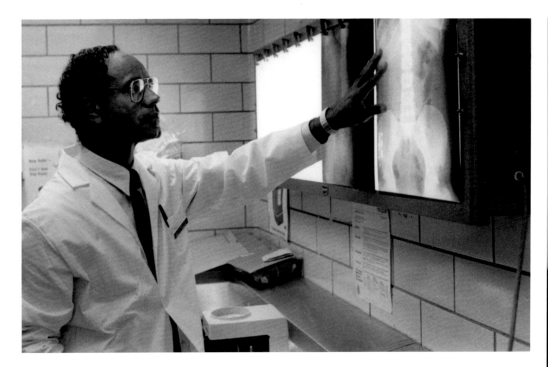

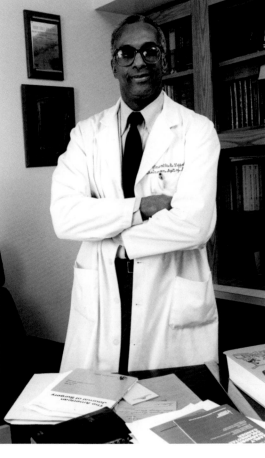

Top left: Dr. Harold Freeman studied the impact of cancer among the poor, and soon the Society, taking its cue from him, began to report on the same and developed programs to confront the problem. Above: Dr. LaSalle D. Leffall, Jr., a surgeon, called on the Society to address the disparities between black and white Americans with regard to cancer prevalence and treatment. In 1978, he was named national president. Opposite right top and bottom: American Cancer Society Hearings on Socio-Economically Disadvantaged, 1989. Opposite far right: Dr. Harold Freeman testifying about the impact of cancer on the poor

are the disenfranchised poor. And they die in greater percentages than their wealthier counterparts.

Following the lead of Dr. Harold Freeman, an African American physician at Harlem Hospital Center, the Society launched an investigation of the impact of cancer on the poor, finding that the thirty-nine million Americans who then lived below the poverty level had a five-year cancer survival rate that was 10 to 15 percent lower than that of wealthier Americans, as well as a higher incidence rate of cancer compared with that of other Americans. Freeman's research was a twist on work that began a decade earlier when the Society made its first effort at righting the racial inequality that existed in its leadership and in its epidemiology focus.

That effort came during the civil rights era and was spurred by two young African Americans, a surgeon named Dr. LaSalle D. Leffall, Jr., and John Henry Jones, the first African American executive hired by the National Home Office. Both men were aware from personal experience that the cancer problems in the black community were different from those among whites. Both wanted to see that gap narrowed. Jones, who worked as an editor and publicist, began to help the Society broaden its perspective and outreach by changing materials so they included blacks, by building a list of black press representatives, and by asking the epidemiology department to begin supplying statistics on cancer among black Americans. Leffall, who began as a volunteer with the Society in the 1960s and was elected national president in 1978, approached it from a crusading researcher's point of view, calling on the Society to "meet the challenge of cancer among black Americans" by focusing attention

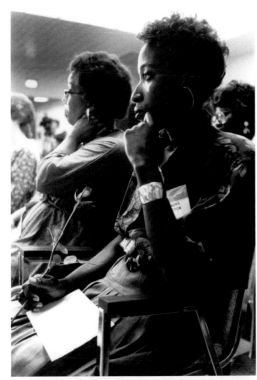

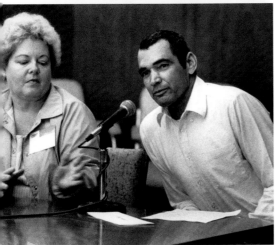

on the disturbing disparities between black and white Americans in cancer prevalence, treatment, and mortality.

Dr. Freeman was asked to testify before a blue-ribbon panel in New York City in 1977 convened by New York Governor Hugh Carey to discuss breast cancer in the state. Freeman had been in Harlem as a surgeon for ten years and had collected information about breast cancer that was, in his words, "very dramatically bad—half of the women were terminal when they walked into the hospital."

At that time, the Society had no presence in Harlem, and Freeman pointed that out. Although the leadership did not like hearing the young doctor's criticisms, they listened and responded by naming him a director at-large of the Society in 1978. "I became a board member from a part of the country that had no representation, no Unit, no Division. There was no way in." Ten years later, the straight-talking doctor was the president of the Society. He had urged the board in 1983 to head up a scholarly study group to gather all the information it could regarding race, poverty, and cancer. Although the recommendation to look beyond just race and at economics was confusing to much of the still heavily white, male, wealthy leadership who'd only just begun to understand the race issue, the Society blessed Freeman's study and made him chair of the subcommittee doing the research.

In 1986, the group published its report, which concluded that who developed cancer and who died was mostly a product of eco-

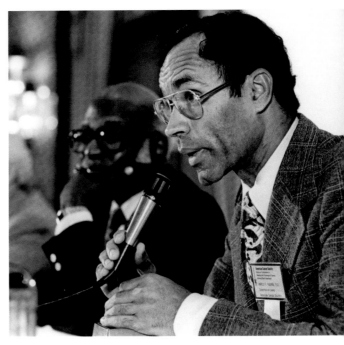

Dr. Harold Freeman testifying

nomics, not just of race. "If that was true, then we had to aim the gun at the poverty issue," Freeman says.

When Dr. Freeman reported his findings at a national press conference, the Society was deluged with letters and calls praising it for taking up the issue of cancer and poverty. During Freeman's presidency, the Society held national hearings on cancer and the poor in seven American cities, ending with a presentation of the report at the White House. Cancer's relationship to poverty, he said, had "become a human issue rather than a racial one, which brought in even more sympathy."

Professional Education

Each of these campaigns was accompanied by an intense effort to alert Americans to their role in shaping their own health, and, at the same time, a companion effort to help educate the medical community about what it needed to be telling patients. The Society has always believed that in order to address its mission of eliminating cancer as a major health problem, there must be a sufficient number of health professionals with knowledge and skills in cancer prevention and control. Originally, the Society was the primary and sometimes the only source of physicians' and nurses' cancer education. In the 1960s, university medical schools began to develop their own programs in oncology, and the focus of the Society's professional education activity shifted from general cancer education to specific oncology education for professionals in areas that have a real impact on cancer prevention and detection—and, thus, on survival.

Virginia Krawiec, MPA, director of health professional training grants, is in charge of the two and a half million dollars in grants handed out each year in what she calls "my little cottage industry." The grants are intended to maintain excellence in cancer prevention and control by supporting individuals in training programs and to provide incentive for people in fields outside oncology to pursue careers in cancer prevention and control. The training grants have been part of the Society since the decision was made in 1946 to develop a research grant program. The first use of the money was to send doctors to Germany to

study radiation therapy being used to treat some tumors, and to teach technicians to read Pap smears, as part of what would become the hugely beneficial area of exfoliative cytology.

The programs were expanded over time into specialty training, such as oncology nursing and social work, and then were expanded again to help influence professionals with an important role in cancer control. Today, a graduate student pursuing a master's degree in oncology nursing can get a stipend of ten thousand dollars for two years; a doctoral candidate may be given a stipend of twenty thousand dollars per year to conduct research on the psychosocial needs of persons with cancer and their families; a primary care physician may receive three years of progressive stipends to develop clinical and teaching expertise to perform independent research or educational innovation in cancer control.

The same rigorous peer-review process used for research grants is applied to the professional training awards; in the last twenty-four years, the Society has received more than fifteen hundred applications and has awarded more than four hundred grants. The Society views its biggest challenge in this area as how best to apply available resources to make the biggest impact. "We have only a small part of the pond here, but we have pretty wide ripples out there," says Krawiec.

❧

Sometimes those ripples are more like waves—and not always ones the Society would like to

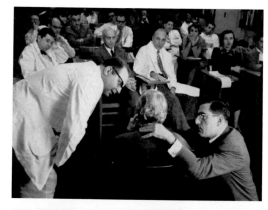

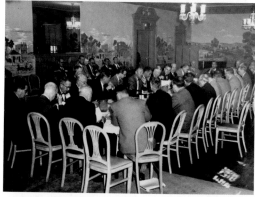

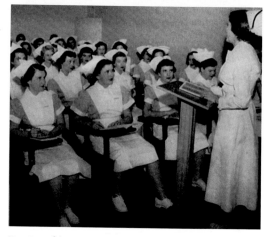

Top: One of the Society's professional education meetings, 1956. Center: Medical and scientific committee at the Society's 1952 Annual Meeting Bottom: Alabama nurses at a cancer seminar Opposite: Peer review for research grants

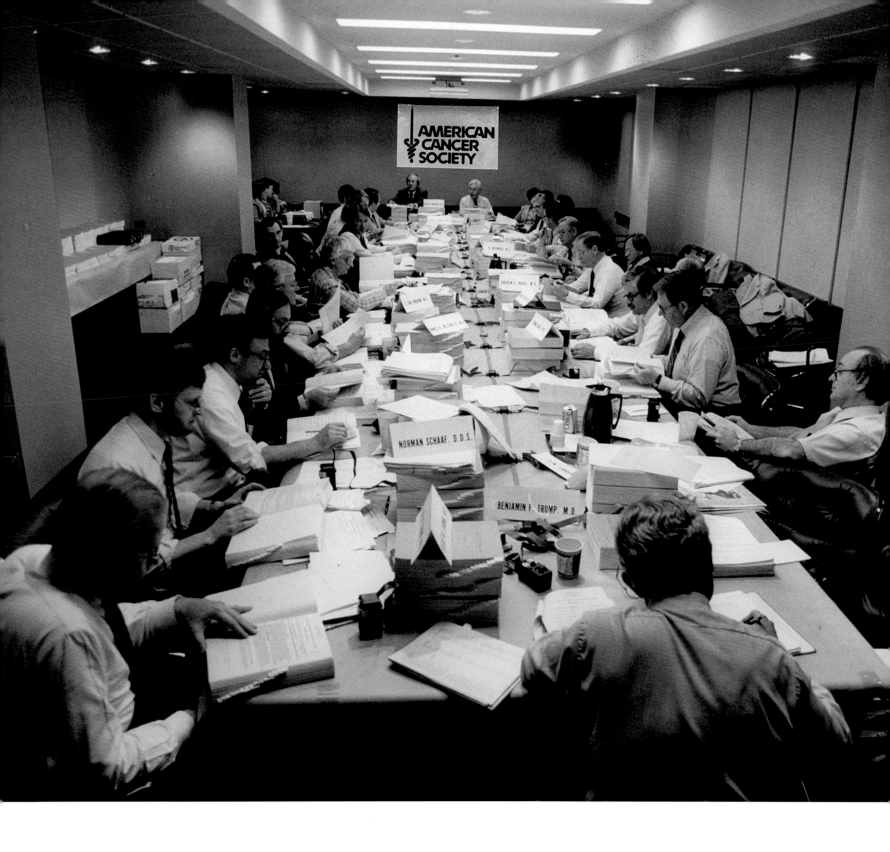

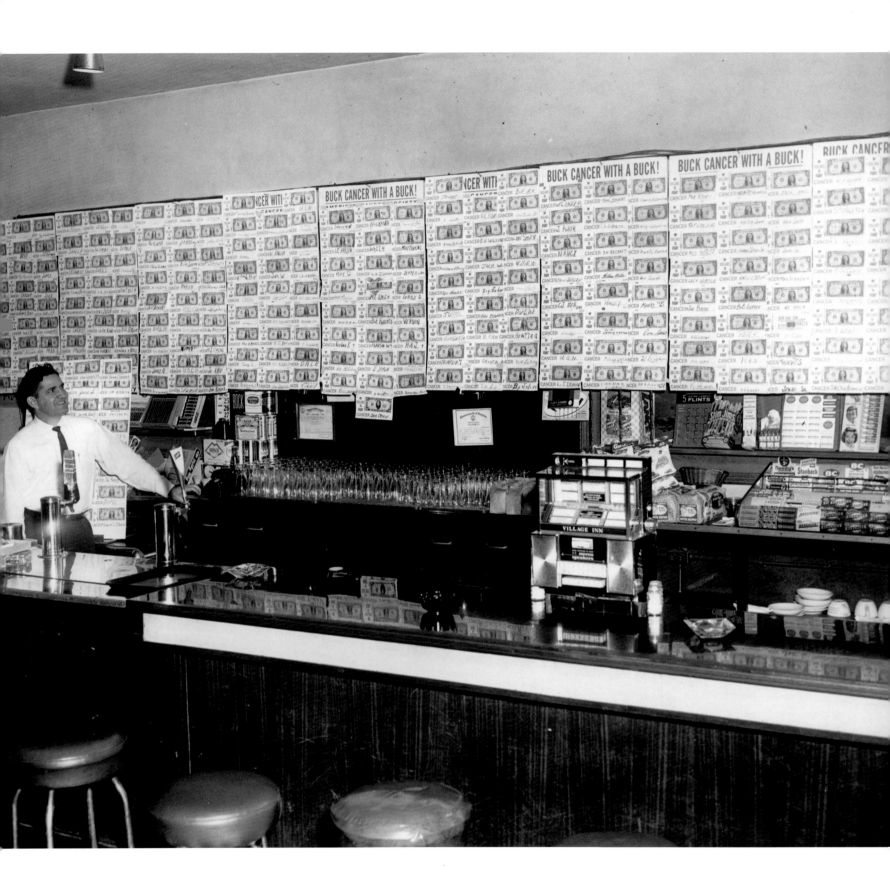

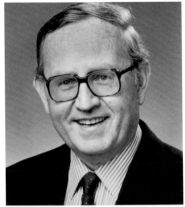

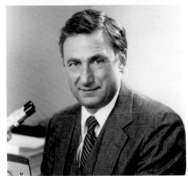

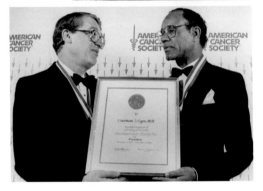

Opposite: During the 1965 Crusade, taverns such as the Village Inn, shown here, raised more than fifteen hundred dollars through the use of Buck Boards provided by the Norfolk–South Norfolk Unit. Top: Dr. Gerald Murphy led the team that discovered the substance PSA, which became the blood test for screening prostate cancer. Center: Dr. David Rosenthal felt more epidemiologic study was required before recommending the PSA test. Above: Dr. Harold Freeman presents an award to Dr. Harmon Eyre. An oncologist from the University of Utah, Eyre became chief medical officer of the Society in 1993. Top right inset: Kathleen Horsch, board chair in 1988, became involved with the Society when a family friend developed cancer.

make. The Society has more than once created controversy with its decisions. Just as the Breast Cancer Detection Demonstration Project gathered criticism, early debate ensued over declaring the prostate-specific antigen (PSA) blood test as the screening test for prostate cancer. The issue was brought to the Society in the mid-1980s by Dr. Gerald Murphy, chief medical officer from 1988 until 1993 and the urological researcher who led the team that discovered the substance PSA.

Dr. David Rosenthal, who became president of the Society in 1998, was one of the lone voices voting against recommending the test to detect cancer. He felt that not enough epidemiologic study had been done at the time of the discussion by the Medical Affairs Committee, and he questioned why, after the problems with mammography, the Society would want to put itself in the same situation again. "I've sat in many rooms where we fought about this," recalls Dr. LaMar McGinnis, a former president and now senior medical consultant with the Society. Rosenthal felt the decision "lost about five years in American cancer leadership." (Today, the recommendation from the Society is that the PSA test should be offered annually beginning at age 50, with testing recommended for men at high risk. The Society advises that information should be provided to the patient so he can make an informed decision.)

Kathleen Horsch

A Personal Battle

The fight against cancer can be very personal. Kathleen "Kay" Horsch, board chair in 1988, first became a volunteer with the Society because a friend's young child had leukemia. Dr. Gordon "Gordy" Klatt spent twenty-four hours walking and running around a Tacoma, Washington, track after he'd treated thousands for cancer over the years and felt the need to do more. Sally West Brooks, RN, MA, chair of the national board in 2006, volunteered with the American Cancer Society at the local, state, and national levels for more than thirty years as a tribute to her mother, a registered nurse who died of breast cancer at age fifty-three.

In the fifteen years they worked together at the helm of the Society, Dr. John Seffrin and Dr. Harmon Eyre seldom forgot the responsibility they carried as the staff leaders in the campaign against cancer. The work is all-consuming.

Both men were volunteers for the Society before they became paid leaders of it. Dr. Eyre was an oncologist and a member of the staff of the University of Utah who was recruited as a volunteer in 1971. His job at the university was to oversee clinical cancer trials and cancer research, and he continually ran into Society volunteers when he would speak in communities without cancer centers. He became national president in 1988,

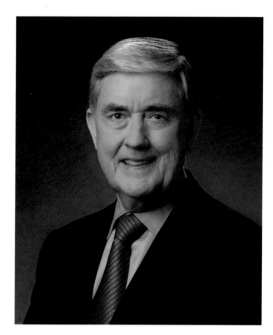

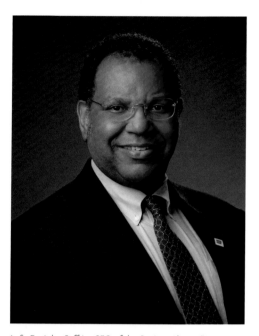

death difference, I had the chance to do it in the cancer area more than any other place."

In late 2007, as Eyre prepared to depart the Society with which he worked for so many years, the Society welcomed Dr. Otis Brawley as its chief medical officer. A world-renowned cancer expert, practicing oncologist, and global leader in the field of health disparities research, Brawley also serves as professor of hematology, oncology, medicine, and epidemiology at Emory University. He had previously served as medical director of the Georgia Cancer Center for Excellence at Grady Memorial Hospital in Atlanta and deputy director for cancer control at Winship Cancer Institute at Emory University. And, like so many others, Dr. Brawley was a volunteer for the Society before joining the staff. And he too embraced the immense, and sometimes all-consuming, responsibility of helping change the face of this disease and move the Society closer to a time without cancer.

five years before he went on to accept the staff position of chief medical officer. Dr. Seffrin was a professor of health education and chair of the Department of Applied Health Science at Indiana University and had started to work with the Society in his home Division in 1976. He became chair of the board in 1990 and 1991 and then took the helm as CEO in 1992.

Both men speak of a greater good in their career choices at the Society: Dr. Eyre came to realize that the number of patients he could personally help in his lifetime was insignificant compared with the number he could affect as the chief medical officer and vice president for research and cancer control for the Society. When Dr. Seffrin was elected chair, he stated, "I came to the realization professionally that if I wanted to make a big difference, a people difference, a life-or-

What brought all these men into the cancer battle and to the Society, and what keeps them and the volunteers with whom they work going, is a sense of urgency. They believe that most of the suffering and dying from cancer today is needless—and that the Society has had and continues to have a huge impact in that area. The Society has had, says Dr. Seffrin, "the institutional wisdom and the courage to fill voids."

They believe that's a battle worth fighting.

The American Cancer Society

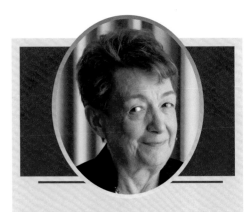

A LASTING LEGACY

Many of the changes in professional education opportunities provided by the American Cancer Society over the last twenty-five years were influenced by Dr. Diane Fink, who was chief mission delivery officer in the California Division of the Society when she died suddenly in 2005. Dr. Fink spearheaded national cancer prevention and education programs and was credited by many with helping decrease the rate of cancer in the United States and improving the quality of life of cancer patients. She was an oncologist at the National Cancer Institute from 1971 to 1981 as a program director for chemotherapy and then director of the division of cancer control and rehabilitation. She had worked for the Society since 1981 in various positions in Atlanta and at the California Division, with an emphasis on promoting cancer control activities for detection, advocacy, prevention, and communication.

Right: Kathy Battle, a child survivor of cancer who became a poster girl for the cancer crusade

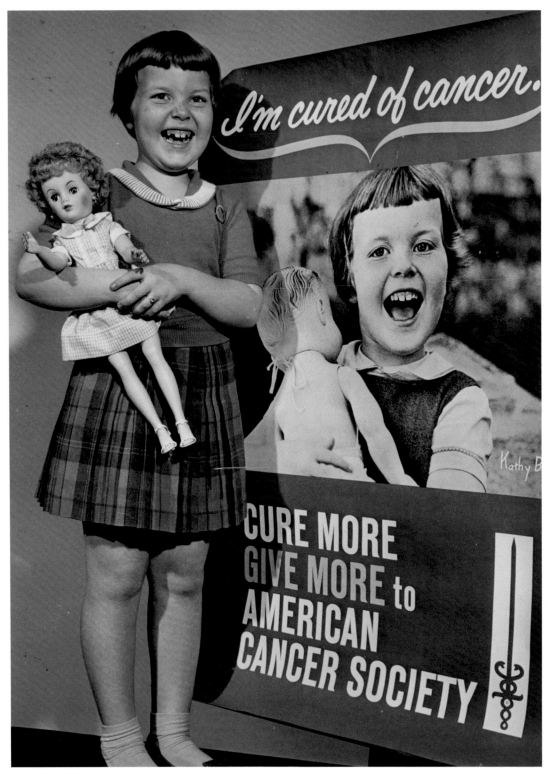

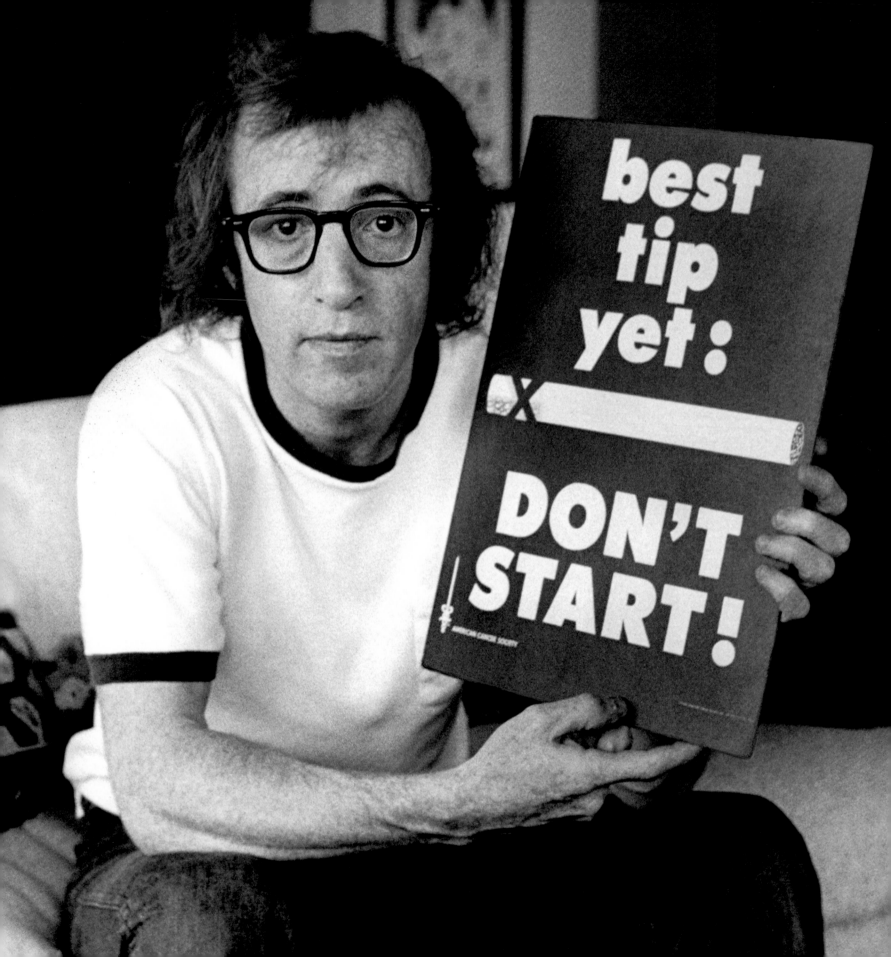

best tip yet: DON'T START!

AMERICAN CANCER SOCIETY

The Tobacco Wars:
Taking on the Killing Machine

They knocked off Joe Camel, the cartoon mascot for Camel cigarettes, in 2000, leaving behind a generation of children who smoked his brand and recognized him more readily than Mickey Mouse. Public outrage killed old Joe, which, if you think about it, is better than what happened to the other great cigarette icon, the Marlboro Man. He just plain died, killed by lung cancer. Among the last words of one of the actors who portrayed the icon were, "Tobacco will kill you, and I'm living proof of it."

Old Joe, an advertising symbol of the R.J. Reynolds tobacco company, and Philip Morris's Marlboro Man were two of the most visible images of a world that embraced cigarettes and smoking as a deadly way to find pleasure, status, or movie-star chic. Together, they helped make their companies the top two tobacco companies in the world and helped convince millions of Americans to smoke their brands. Meanwhile, the companies hid what they knew about tobacco—that it was addictive and could be made more so with additives. Together, they denied culpability as hundreds of thousands of their customers died of smoking-induced diseases.

The situation was enough to launch one of the American Cancer Society's most important crusades: what is now more than

Opposite: Woody Allen is one of many celebrities who has volunteered their services to the American Cancer Society.

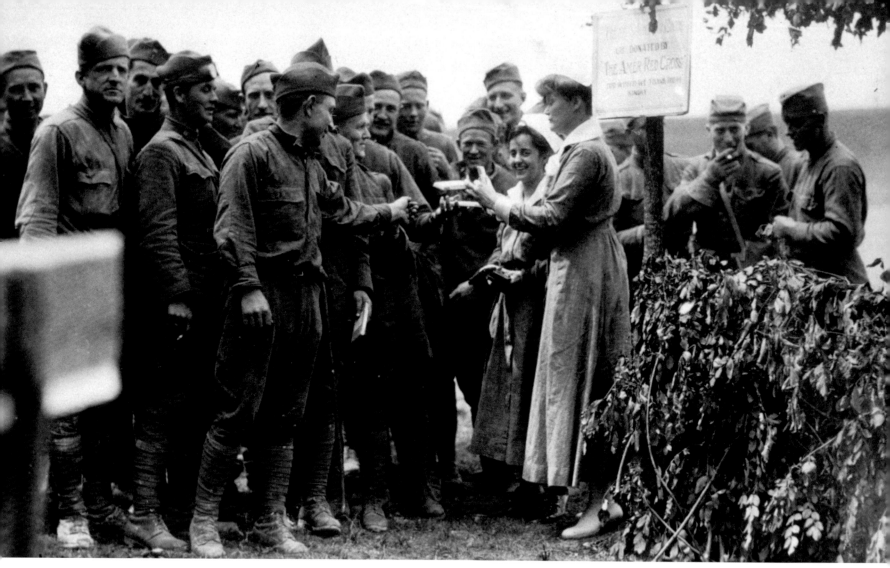

fifty years of work to stop death at the end of a burning cigarette.

Dr. E. Cuyler Hammond couldn't have known the firestorm he was setting off when he began a puzzled search through numbers that showed an unsettling trend in the health of Americans in the 1930s and 1940s. Dr. Hammond was the director of statistical research at the Society, hired to study the effectiveness of Society programs and to track statistics from cancer diagnosis through death.

He found a curious thing. Lung cancer deaths, once so rare that a medical school professor talked of the "once in a lifetime" opportunity to see a case in an autopsy in 1919, were becoming all too common. Doctors who'd never seen a single case in years of medical practice were suddenly seeing clusters of cases—one reporting eight cases in six months, all men who'd begun smoking in World War I, when cigarettes were first distributed to soldiers, unknowingly, by the American Red Cross and the Young Men's Christian Association. There

Above: Free cigarettes were passed out to World War I soldiers. Years later, studies demonstrated a sharp spike in cancer-related deaths among war veterans.

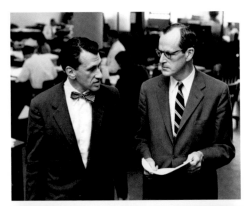

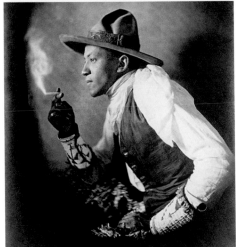

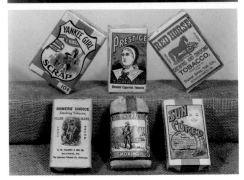

Top: Dr. E. Cuyler Hammond (right) charted a 700 percent increase in lung cancer cases among men in the 1930s and 1940s. Like his colleague Dr. Daniel Horn, pictured with him, Hammond was himself a veteran and a chain smoker. Center: Cowboys, soldiers, doctors . . . any role model would do for the cigarette industry. Bottom: Some early cigarette brands

were 2,400 lung cancer deaths reported in the United States in 1928; by 1948, that number was up to 16,331—almost a 700 percent increase.

Until the boom years of World War I—when cigarette production increased from under ten billion a year to nearly seventy billion a year—most smokers were men, and most chose cigars or pipes. Cigarette smoking was considered pedestrian and unmanly, a dirty little sin that women hid and men considered a sign of cheapness, according to Thomas Addison, MD, a clinical professor of medicine at the University of California at San Francisco who published a tobacco chronology in 1998.

When the American boys came back from the war, though, they had a swagger in their hips and cigarettes dangling from their lips—and a habit the cigarette industry was eager to feed. Everyone wanted their smokes—housewives, lawyers, steel mill workers, and doctors. In 1927, the American Tobacco Company began a campaign claiming that 11,105 physicians endorsed Lucky Strikes as "less irritating to sensitive or tender throats than any other cigarettes." By 1934, the American Medical Association was accepting tobacco advertising in its journals. By 1948, after the Second World War, in which the Red Cross gave out free cigarettes to the fighting men and women, "the golden age of tobacco advertising was upon us," Addison reported.

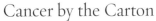

Soldiers, following the war, came home smoking.

Edward R. Murrow never appeared on television without his cigarette, Humphrey Bogart enjoyed his Camels in Rick's Café Américain in *Casablanca*, and movie-star pinup Rita Hayworth was pledging fealty to Chesterfields in print ads that swore, "In my case, it's Chesterfield." Hammond, out of the military and just starting his new job at the Society in 1947, was a three-pack-a-day man; his assistant, Dr. Daniel Horn, smoked along with him, enjoying that "cooling sensation of menthol" from Kools and that "fine tobacco" from Lucky Strikes.

The nation was hooked on what the cigarette industry in a full-page advertisement in 448 newspapers called the "solace, relaxation and enjoyment to mankind" that only they were able to give the world.

Unfortunately, America would discover there was a price to pay for all that enjoyment.

Cancer by the Carton

There had long been talk that smoking might cause health problems. One of the first observations linking tobacco and cancer was made in 1916 by Dr. Frederick Hoffman, an early cancer epidemiologist and one of the founders of the Society. Speaking at a conference in New Orleans, Dr. Hoffman pointed out the relationship between the use of tobacco and the increased risk of throat and mouth cancer. This observation went

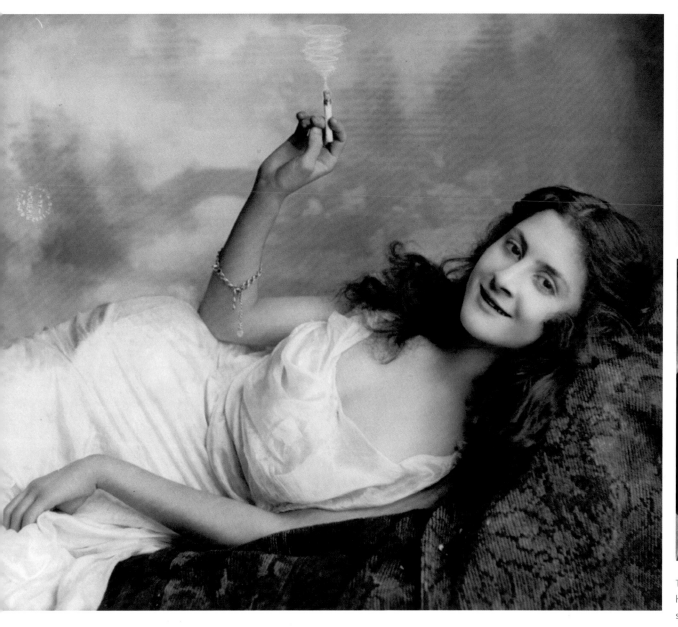

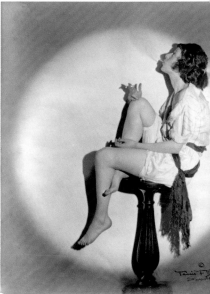

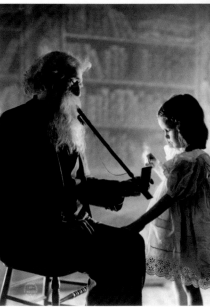

This page and opposite: Photos showing how early on, film and media depicted smoking as glamorous, as well as a way to set a tone or express a feeling or emotion.

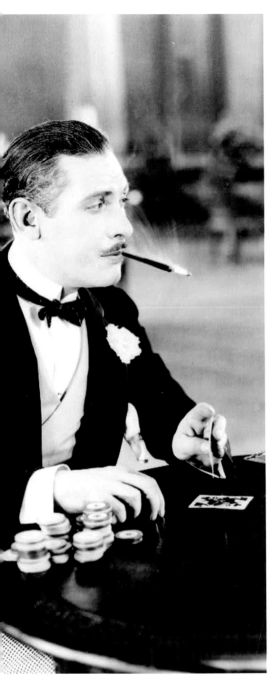

unheeded for years and was all but forgotten. Years later, four important studies were published in America in 1950 on the smoking habits of people with lung cancer as compared with people free of the disease; two similar ones, also showing a correlation between smoking and lung cancer, were published two years later in England.

In December 1952, *Reader's Digest* reprinted a two-page article titled "Cancer by the Carton." The article, which had appeared in an earlier newsletter, accused the tobacco industry of covering up the link between tobacco and lung cancer. With a circulation of seven million, the *Digest* was the top-selling magazine in America. It took no advertising at the time, which allowed it to publish the controversial article without fear of losing advertising revenue. The article jolted America. Similar reports began appearing in other national magazines, and cigarette sales declined in America for the first time since the Great Depression.

Although the evidence that smoking was associated with lung cancer was compelling, it was not scientifically conclusive. Hammond knew about these reports but had deep doubts about the validity of studies implicating cigarettes. He told a reporter that he believed the people who had interviewed the lung cancer patients probably induced an emotional bias that led them to make suspicious confessions of heavy smoking. But clearly something was happening. Acting on data that showed lung cancer rising at an alarming rate, Hammond began to systematically examine common factors. He finally concluded that the increase might be caused by the inhalation of fumes from one of three things: oil, tar, or cigarettes.

Hammond realized he needed some sort of super-sized "prospective" study—following people in the future, not just looking at current numbers—to form a scientifically accurate opinion. He had never seen a study of this sort done and knew of no experts who could do it. When he asked the Gallup and Roper polling organizations how much it would cost, they estimated a cost of five million dollars for the initial interviews alone. Hammond intended to screen two hundred fifty thousand men, and he wanted the men followed for five years. The cost would probably balloon to ten million dollars, and neither Roper nor Gallup knew how to trace a couple of hundred thousand people for years. It had never been done.

The leadership of the Society was already dubious about the whole idea, far from convinced about the possibility of a causal relationship between cigarettes and lung cancer. Besides their scientific doubts, the board members had political ones. The tobacco industry was extremely powerful, involving itself in almost every aspect of American business. It even had its tentacles in the Society, primarily in its Southern Divisions, where most of the tobacco was grown and where thousands of volunteers relied on the tobacco industry for jobs. Even Mary

Lasker had ties to the industry: her husband, Albert, had handled the American Tobacco Company's Lucky Strikes account at his advertising company during the 1920s and 1930s, targeting women with ads that included the famous message to "Reach for a Lucky instead of a sweet" to establish an association between smoking and slimness.

Dr. Charles Cameron, a heavy smoker and the medical director of the Society, backed Hammond, although he also expressed doubts that smoking was tied to lung cancer. Prominent board members Elmer Bobst and Dr. Alton Ochsner were both pushing for the study. Dr. Ochsner, the chief of surgery at Tulane University and president of the Society in 1950, had told the International Cancer Congress in 1939 that he thought cigarettes were causing the disease after he began to see man after man with lung cancer.

The board ultimately decided to let Hammond launch the research project. However, because of the enormous expense, the project was put on hold until financial support for it could be found, which everyone acknowledged might take quite a trick.

It was Dr. Hammond's wife, Marian, who made an innovative suggestion of enormous importance: since the Society had such a vast network of volunteers—many of them

Lawrence Garfinkel

well-educated women who had ended their professional careers when they married—why not use the volunteers to conduct the study? The Society endorsed the plan, despite continued reservations about the study itself. A young cancer researcher, Lawrence Garfinkel, MA, joined the project with Drs. Hammond and Horn and designed the study questionnaire. Several small pilot projects were conducted to perfect and refine the study. Preliminary data from the pilots verified that the project was feasible and could obtain reliable and useful data. Twenty-seven hundred volunteers in nine states were recruited and trained, and the first Cancer Prevention Study (CPS I) was launched in 1952.

The volunteers were asked to do an initial interview and then check the list of persons enrolled every November for five years and report whether the persons were alive or dead. If they had died, Hammond and Horn asked the health departments in each state to give them a copy of the death certificate showing cause of death. All this information was entered by hand onto the bewildering file cards of a primitive keypunch machine that Hammond, Horn, and Garfinkel used to collate information card by card. The volunteers did their jobs well, going to extraordinary lengths to get in touch with "their" patients. The information they

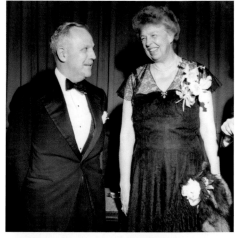

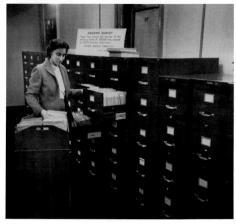

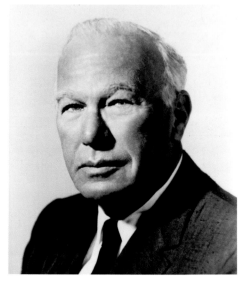

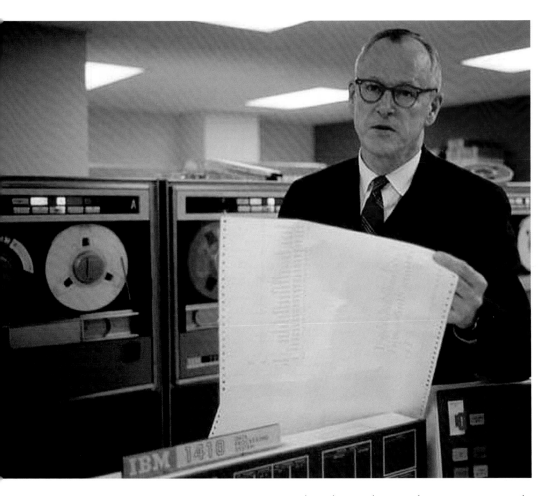

Opposite inset: Lawrence Garfinkel designed the study questionnaire for the Cancer Prevention Study—and promptly gave up smoking upon seeing the results. Opposite top right: As early as 1939, Dr. Alton Ochsner (shown here at a function with Eleanor Roosevelt) had asserted that cigarettes were causing cancer. Opposite center: A woman from the American Cancer Society grabbing files of questionnaires that charted lung cancer in smokers. Opposite bottom: Elmer Bobst was a prominent board member who pushed for the first Cancer Prevention Study. Above: Dr. E. Cuyler Hammond was the first to realize the need for a broad-scale "prospective" study on lung cancer—a study that tracked future statistics, not numbers from the present or past.

the study was complete and a full year before he had expected to have any significant findings. He told the doctors—all those doctors with cigarettes in their front pockets—that cigarette smokers from fifty to seventy years of age had a death rate that was as much as 75 percent higher than nonsmokers. He told them that the smokers had higher incidences of oral cancers. And he told them that cigarette smokers had twice as many coronary heart attacks as non-smokers. Explaining why he had rushed to get the information out, he said, "We found cigarette smokers had so much higher death rates that we didn't think we should withhold the information another year."

Hammond had every reason to feel the weight of his findings: by 1955, lung cancer was responsible for approximately one in eighteen deaths among men.

When the *Journal of the American Medical Association* (*JAMA*) published the final report by Hammond and Horn in 1958, the results confirmed that the risk of lung cancer death was nine times greater for smokers than for nonsmokers. The risk was also directly related to the number of cigarettes smoked per day. Previous smokers who stopped using tobacco enjoyed a lower risk, but never the same as that of someone who never smoked. Pipe smokers had a lower risk than cigarette smokers and higher than nonsmokers.

Big Tobacco Fights Back

The tobacco industry did not go quietly into the night.

gathered was clean and precise; upon early review of the data at two years, 97 percent of the forms submitted were acceptable and valid for review and statistical analysis.

That's when Hammond, Horn, and Garfinkel all gave up smoking.

The numbers were stupefying: what they were seeing was an epidemic of death that could only be attributable to smoking. Hammond broke standard scientific procedures and asked to address the American Medical Association's annual convention in San Francisco in June 1954, three years before

Although the report generated headlines all over the world, cigarette sales showed only a brief downturn and rebounded forcefully the next year. In the meantime, the tobacco companies coughed up their newest offering to smokers, filtered cigarettes that promised "real health protection." Philip Morris introduced the "Tattooed Man" campaign in 1955, showing the image of the "new Marlboro smoker as a lean, relaxed outdoorsman . . . whose tattooed wrist suggested a romantic past . . . [and] who merited respect," as *Esquire* magazine described it. The Tattooed Man ultimately became the Marlboro Man, and Marlboro became the top-selling filtered cigarette in New York.

After *JAMA* published Hammond and Horn's final report in 1958 linking tobacco smoking to lung cancer and many related diseases, the tobacco industry tried to obfuscate the results by forming the Tobacco Industry Research Committee (later called the Council for Tobacco Research). The committee's function was to develop research invalidating the Society's study and other scientific reports that showed the risk of cancer to smokers. The committee even went so far as to prepare secret reports on key members of the Society, looking for ways to discredit them.

Emerson Foote, who had continued to guide the Society's public relations efforts after he helped in the reorganization in 1946, was the subject of one such report, which suggested that members of the Tobacco Institute board should read a popular book called *The Hucksters*. Foote, a successful New York advertising whiz,

had publicly attacked tobacco advertising while his agency was handling twenty million dollars in cigarette billings. His decision to drop the twelve-million-dollar American Tobacco Company account in 1948 made headlines. Although the book about the Madison Avenue advertising agency was fiction, one of the main characters was supposed to be Foote. Perhaps, the Tobacco Institute report suggested, a "reading or re-reading of this novel . . . could be a helpful source of information."

Years later, papers from the Tobacco Institute would be used in a two-hundred-eighty-billion-dollar federal lawsuit against Big Tobacco. Among other items, these papers revealed payments to scientists under a covert "scientific witness" program used to refute the negative reports emerging on the impact of cigarette smoking. One of the people first hired by the Tobacco Industry Research Committee, to the chagrin of the Society's leadership, was Dr. Clarence Cook Little, former managing director of the Society. According to Richard Kluger's Pulitzer Prize–winning book on the tobacco industry, the Society's medical director Charles Cameron "thought that Little 'must have been pretty hard up' and that his accepting the new position was 'purely a mercenary kind of thing,' to survive financially in his old age. Whatever the reason, Cameron added 'Nobody at the society admired him for it.'"

The debate over cigarettes raged for four years, both in the boardroom of the Society and in the outside world, after

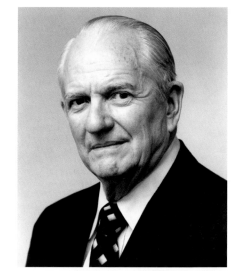

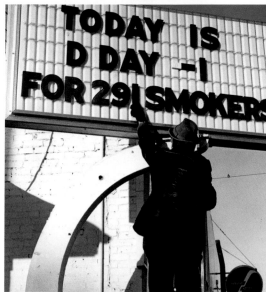

Top: Emerson Foote. Bottom: A Minnesota weekly made national news with its "Don't Smoke" Day on January 7, 1974. The prime force behind the D-Day Campaign was Lynn Smith, publisher of the *Monticello Times*, who had been active in the Minnesota Division of the Society and who had quit smoking in 1954. Opposite: Dr. Luther Terry, former U.S. Surgeon General, and Senator Robert Kennedy, who addressed the participants at the 1967 World Conference on Smoking and Health

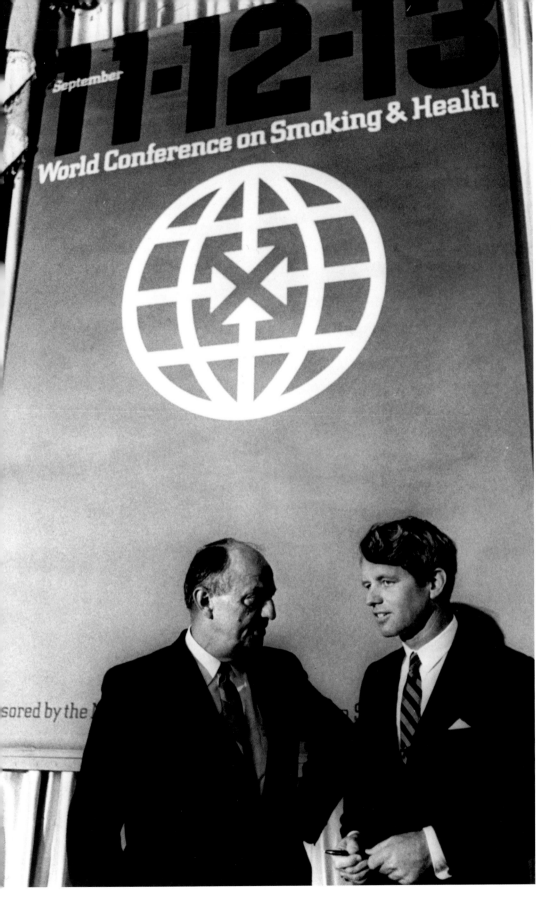

Hammond and Horn made their initial report to the AMA. Finally, in 1958, faced with the publication of its own study, the board voted overwhelmingly for a strong statement against smoking. It still stood very much alone; the federal government had suppressed a surgeon general's report for two years, finally releasing a watered-down version in 1959. A subsequent editorial in *JAMA* stated only that there were not enough facts to clearly state that smoking caused cancer.

However, the Society grew increasingly alarmed by the rising diagnoses and death toll from lung cancer and other respiratory and heart problems. In 1960, it voted to publish a report warning the American public about the risk of lung cancer from tobacco use, stating "beyond a reasonable doubt" that cigarette smoking was the major cause of lung cancer. A year later, three influential health organizations—the American Heart Association, the American Public Health Association, and the National Tuberculosis Association (now the American Lung Association)—joined the Society in beseeching President John F. Kennedy to appoint a commission to look into the widespread implications of the tobacco problem. It was a precarious move for all the organizations, because it meant they had entered the risky arena of politics—while directly aligning themselves against one of the wealthiest and most powerful industries in America.

A month later, Surgeon General Luther K. Terry announced he was appointing a medical and scientific committee to undertake a comprehensive review of all data on smoking and health. The committee of ten expert physicians took fourteen months to study eleven hundred research reports on smoking and health and a summary of six thousand other studies.

The surgeon general's report, released in 1964, declared cigarette smoking to be "a health hazard of sufficient import in the U.S. to warrant appropriate remedial action." Working on that report was a key member of the Surgeon General's Advisory Committee on Smoking and Health, Dr. Charles A. LeMaistre. He was later to become the Society's national president in 1986. Throughout his career, which included eighteen years as president of the University of Texas M. D. Anderson Cancer Center, LeMaistre actively promoted efforts to increase public awareness of smoking risks. The report unleashed a tide of political, medical, and corporate controversy that still has ramifications today; since then, the surgeon general's office has released twenty-eight more reports on the consequences of smoking. At the same time, the Society's public stand against the use of tobacco ushered in a new era for the organization, one marked by advocacy for public policies that protect Americans from cancer (see Chapter 9, "Powerful Friends"). The release of the 1964 report also clearly drew the battle lines between the Society and Big Tobacco.

A Billion Reasons to Fight

The letter from the Cleveland lawyer to the New York lawyer used words you wouldn't

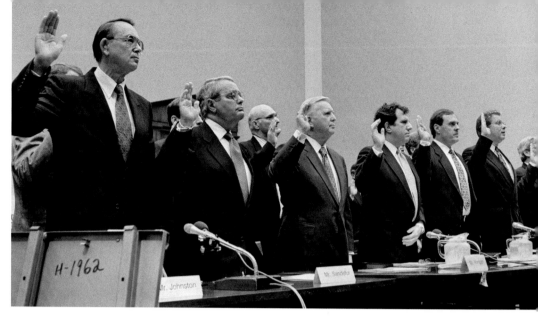

Above: In 1994, chairmen from seven leading tobacco companies testified before Congress. Here, the executives are sworn in before the House Subcommittee on Health and the Environment. All would testify that they believed nicotine was not addictive.

expect to see in a letter about two scientists—"attack," "ambush," "specious allegations," "scurrilous accusations"—three single-spaced typed pages that ended with a demand for an apology. But Dr. Michael Thun had learned that the business he is in—overseeing, producing, and explaining findings in the Society's epidemiology department, particularly around smoking—is a ferocious one. "You take a lot of knocks in the process."

The letter was written in 1995 after Dr. Thun, vice president for epidemiology and surveillance research, crossed swords briefly at a professional conference with a scientist on the payroll of the Tobacco Institute. The tobacco researcher, Dr. Maurice LeVois, gave a presentation about environmental tobacco smoke (ETS, also known as secondhand smoke) using information extracted from two Society studies, Cancer Prevention Studies (CPS) I and II. Thun, hearing about the report the day LeVois was to give it, asked for two minutes to rebut some of the report. The epidemiolo-

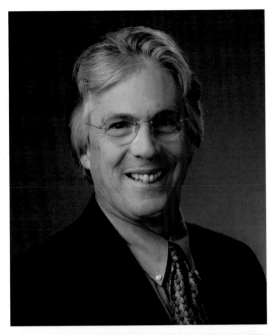

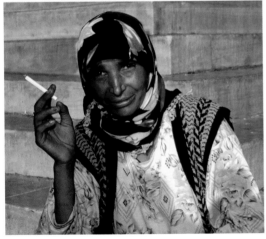

Top: Dr. Michael Thun. Bottom: Increasingly, the burden of deaths caused by cigarette smoking falls on poor and developing countries.

gist had twice before seen the tobacco industry misuse data from the reports, and he wanted those two minutes to set the record straight.

The letter complaining about his scandalous behavior arrived two weeks later. Dr. Thun was dumbfounded. He puzzled over it for days, trying to figure out why the scientist and the lawyer had reacted so strongly. He puzzled right through the three-page response from the Society's own attorney ("vituperative," "grossly inaccurate," "unfounded personal attacks"). He puzzled right through his preparations as a witness in a case the state of Mississippi had brought against the tobacco industry for reimbursement of Medicaid and Medicare payments to people with tobacco-induced cancers.

His puzzling stopped there. "I guess they wanted to show me as a fanatic, to discredit me when I got on the stand," the most unfanatical Thun realized.

The clash between the Society and Big Tobacco over America's health is an open one, seldom hidden from public view. What began as purely a scientific exercise has become a full-scale fight, with the Society helping to marshal troops and weapons against the multibillion-dollar tobacco industry. The stakes are high: the American Cancer Society reports that cigarettes killed one hundred million people in the twentieth century, a significant number of them Americans. Thun estimates that cigarettes will kill one billion in the twenty-first centu-

ry—with the burden of death increasingly falling on poor people in developing countries. As the number of cigarettes sold in the United States has decreased, the number sold in countries such as China, Mexico, and the former Soviet Union, where there are few restrictions, have surged. "The industry is effectively a cancer itself that draws its nutrients from developing countries," he says.

Despite the tremendous advocacy efforts in this country—including efforts to create smoke-free cities and states, warning labels on every pack of cigarettes, advertising bans, increased tools to help smokers overcome their addictions, and the continued development of more epidemiologic information showing just how deadly smoking is—one in five Americans still smoke today, and many more overseas will smoke tomorrow. The Society sees it as its moral obligation to reduce the number of smokers as much as possible. As Big Tobacco has lost some of its grip on America and has set its sights on foreign countries, the Society has become increasingly active in the global fight against cigarettes and smoking through its association with the International Union Against Cancer (UICC), the world's largest independent, nonprofit, nongovernmental association of cancer-fighting organizations.

❧

Yet, sometimes it seems that tobacco is a two-headed dragon.

Following the surgeon general's report in 1964, Big Tobacco began to push filters and low-tar cigarettes, including evidence claiming that some of the tars—one of the cancer-causing elements in tobacco—could be filtered out. Smoking robots designed to test the amount of tar going into the body were used to demonstrate how much tar the filters were removing, and Americans were assured that this "breakthrough" in cigarette manufacturing would allow them to continue to smoke without risk. In 1989, twenty-five years after the government had issued its original report on smoking, the surgeon general prepared a progress report and asked the Society to supply epidemiologic information based on CPS I and II.

When the Society's scientists began to look at the data, they made what Thun calls the "shocking disclosure" that cancer risks had increased since the introduction of filtered cigarettes. At first, he said, no one knew what to think of this finding: the robots had shown a reduction in the amount of cancer-causing tar that would go into the body. The scientists eventually came to two realizations. The first was that machines don't actually measure what smokers inhale. Smoking is driven by the need to satisfy the nicotine addiction; if you reduce the amount of nicotine in each cigarette, smokers will inhale more deeply or smoke more. You could fool the machine but never the smoker about how much tar and nicotine were going into the body. Tar and nicotine aren't

all that go into the body when cigarettes are burning—so do more than four thousand chemicals, at least sixty-nine of them known carcinogens, and any number of the almost six hundred additives allowed in the manufacture of cigarettes.

The other realization was that how long a person had smoked was far more important than the number of cigarettes smoked each day. Men, who had started smoking in waves before their female peers, showed a doubled increase in risk between 1959 and 1989. But now women, targeted through intense marketing studies and lured in by slogans such as Virginia Slims' "We've come a long way, Baby," campaign were showing their own epidemic of death.

This last finding spurred the surgeon general to produce a report in 1990 on the health benefits of smoking cessation—and has helped reduce the level of smoking in America to what it was in World War II. Among the states registering the lowest percentage of smokers is California, which led the grassroots revolt against smoking, with the help of the American Cancer Society.

David and Goliath

In the late 1980s, a group of California citizens decided something had to be done in their trendsetting state to further reduce smoking. Restaurants smelled like smoke, teenagers were buying into the cigarette culture at alarming rates, and people were dying. The group had already been trying for several

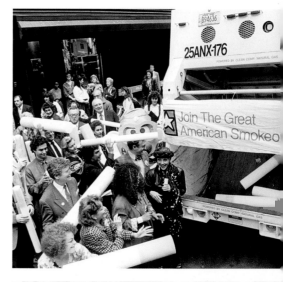

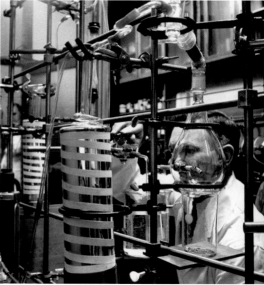

Top: The Great American Smokeout® is but one of several programs developed over the years to encourage people to quit smoking. Bottom: A chemist of the American Tobacco Company studying the effects of smoking cigarettes on a smoking machine. Opposite: Senator Edward Kennedy introduces tobacco control legislation the day before the Great American Smokeout, 1989.

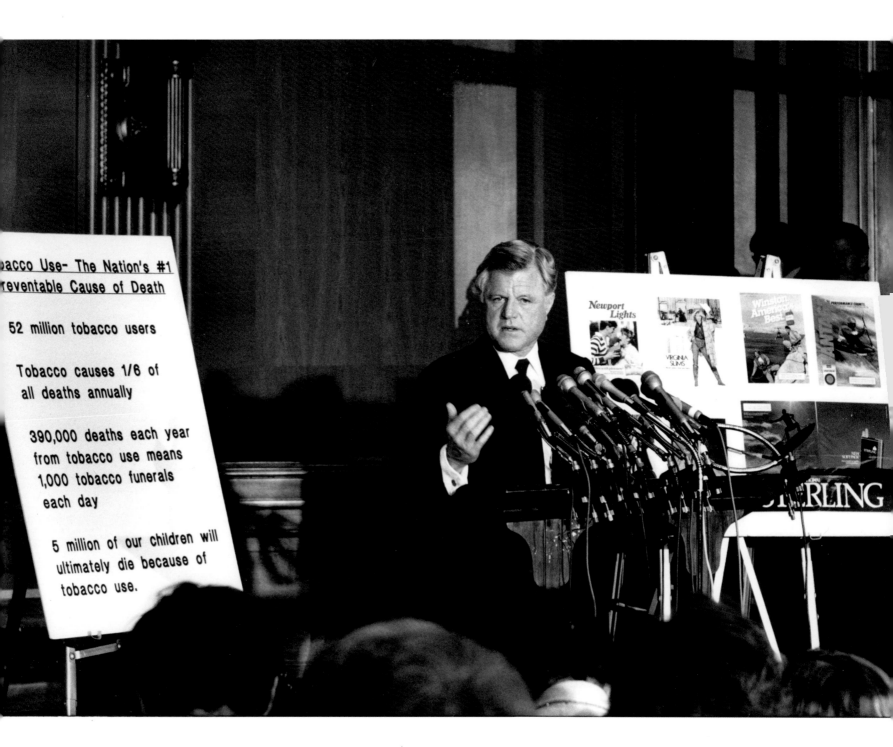

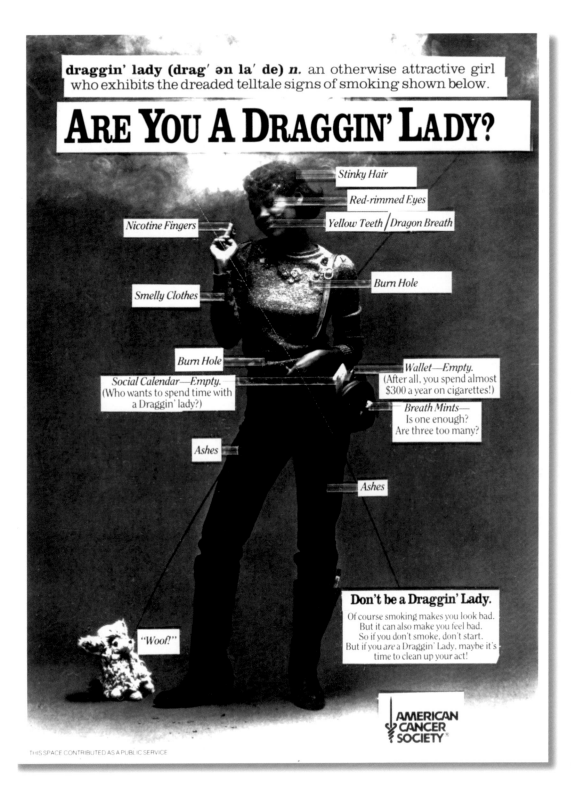

draggin' lady (drag′ ən la′ de) n. an otherwise attractive girl who exhibits the dreaded telltale signs of smoking shown below.

ARE YOU A DRAGGIN' LADY?

Stinky Hair

Red-rimmed Eyes

Yellow Teeth / Dragon Breath

Nicotine Fingers

Burn Hole

Smelly Clothes

Burn Hole

Social Calendar—Empty.
(Who wants to spend time with a Draggin' lady?)

Wallet—Empty.
(After all, you spend almost $300 a year on cigarettes!)

Breath Mints—
Is one enough?
Are three too many?

Ashes

Ashes

"Woof!"

Don't be a Draggin' Lady.
Of course smoking makes you look bad.
But it can also make you feel bad.
So if you don't smoke, don't start.
But if you *are* a Draggin' Lady, maybe it's time to clean up your act!

AMERICAN CANCER SOCIETY

THIS SPACE CONTRIBUTED AS A PUBLIC SERVICE

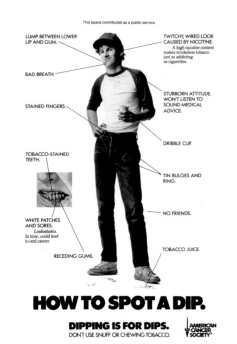

This space contributed as a public service.

LUMP BETWEEN LOWER LIP AND GUM.

TWITCHY, WIRED LOOK CAUSED BY NICOTINE.
A high nicotine content makes smokeless tobacco just as addicting as cigarettes.

BAD BREATH.

STAINED FINGERS.

STUBBORN ATTITUDE. WON'T LISTEN TO SOUND MEDICAL ADVICE.

TOBACCO-STAINED TEETH.

DRIBBLE CUP.

TIN BULGES AND RING.

NO FRIENDS.

WHITE PATCHES AND SORES.
Leukoplakia.
In time, could lead to oral cancer.

RECEDING GUMS.

TOBACCO JUICE.

HOW TO SPOT A DIP.

DIPPING IS FOR DIPS.
DON'T USE SNUFF OR CHEWING TOBACCO.

AMERICAN CANCER SOCIETY

Ad No. 1287-K (7" x 10")
Created as a public service by
N W Ayer/SF

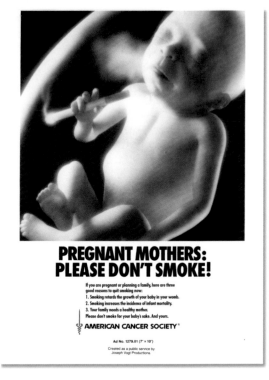

PREGNANT MOTHERS: PLEASE DON'T SMOKE!

If you are pregnant or planning a family, here are three good reasons to quit smoking now:
1. Smoking retards the growth of your baby in your womb.
2. Smoking increases the incidence of infant mortality.
3. Your family needs a healthy mother.
Please don't smoke for your baby's sake. And yours.

AMERICAN CANCER SOCIETY

Ad No. 1279.01 (7" × 10")
Created as a public service by
Joseph Vogt Productions.

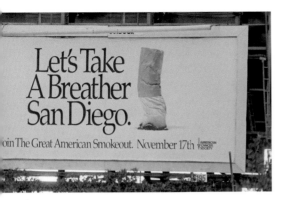

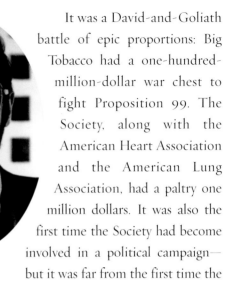
Dr. Dileep G. Bal

Opposite: American Cancer Society ads that appeared in the 1980s. Top: Great American Smokeout® billboard. Below: Dr. C. Everett Koop, surgeon general, and Dr. Charles A. LeMaistre, at a joint news conference of the American Cancer Society, the American Heart Association, and the American Lung Association, in which Dr. Koop called upon the coalition to be the first to join him and take up the challenge for a "smoke-free society by the year 2000." Right inset: Dr. Dileep G. Bal, a California health official and Society volunteer, helped organize what became known as Proposition 99—a steep tax on cigarettes sold in the state.

years to get a decent tobacco control program through a state legislature heavily dependent on tobacco money to support politics as usual. Finally, the Society and others in the public health care arena, including Dr. Dileep G. Bal, chief of the cancer control branch within the California Department of Health Services and a longtime volunteer (who would later become the Society's president in 2001), organized a petition drive to put an initiative on the November 1988 ballot to place a twenty-five-cent tax on each pack of cigarettes sold in the state. The California Tobacco Health Protection Act of 1988, also known as Proposition 99, was born.

It was a David-and-Goliath battle of epic proportions: Big Tobacco had a one-hundred-million-dollar war chest to fight Proposition 99. The Society, along with the American Heart Association and the American Lung Association, had a paltry one million dollars. It was also the first time the Society had become involved in a political campaign—but it was far from the first time the tobacco industry had played politics.

Against all odds, California voters in November 1988 approved Proposition 99. The tax increase would bring in about six hundred fifty million dollars that could be earmarked for programs to reduce smoking, provide health care services to indigent citizens, support tobacco-related research, and fund resource programs for the environment. But the battle was far from over.

Dr. Bal's budget as head of the state's cancer control branch was only two hundred fifty thousand dollars. With the passage of Proposition 99, his annual budget grew to one hundred million. Maddeningly, the legislature, still bending to Big Tobacco for campaign contributions, wouldn't release the money that was now coming into state coffers from the new tax. "The whole thing became so obscene politically that the papers came out strongly against the legislature being the butt of the cigarette industry,"

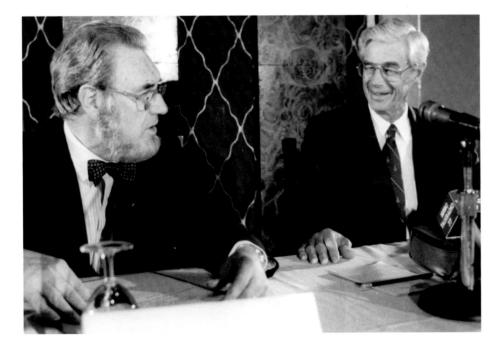

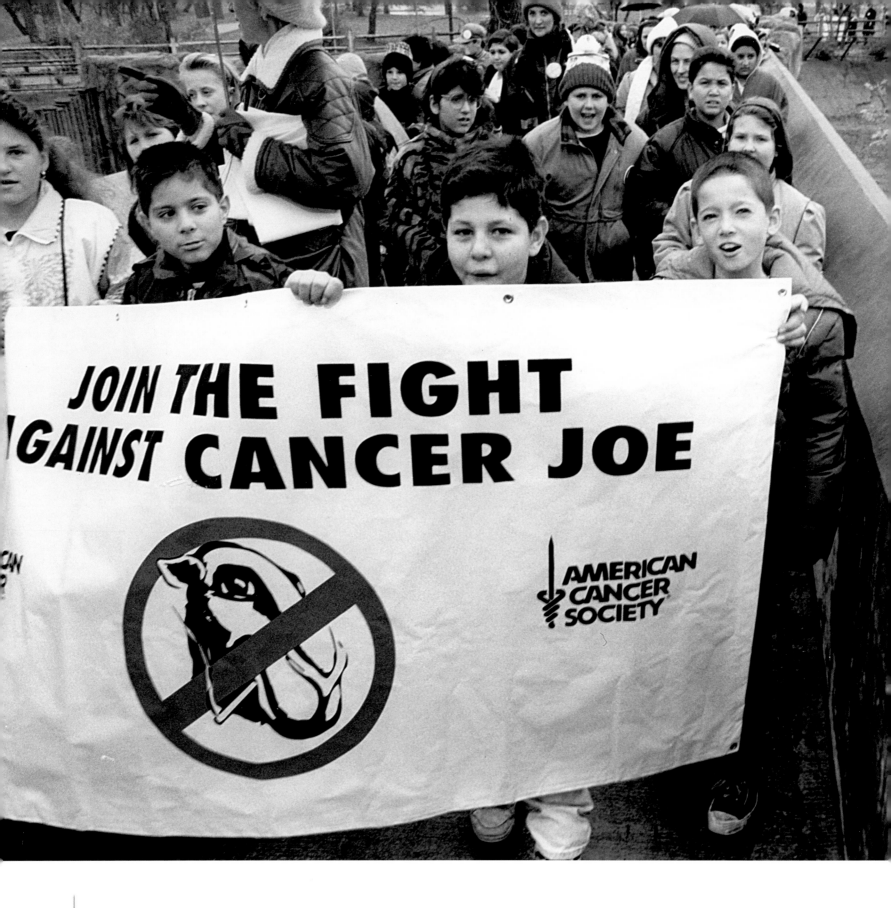

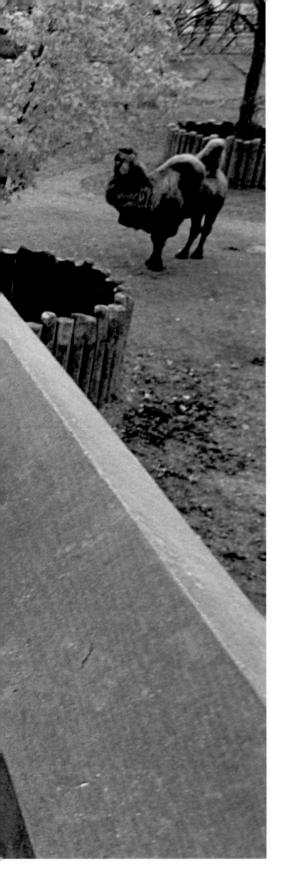

Left: The Illinois Division rallied a thousand Chicago-area fifth-graders at the Lincoln Park Zoo to learn about real camels, who don't shoot pool, smoke cigarettes, or wear leather.

JOE CAMEL

The R.J. Reynolds Company introduced Camel cigarettes in 1913. The camel on the front of the package was based on a circus camel named "Old Joe" that distributed free cigarettes as it paraded through towns.

In 1988 "Joe Camel," a cartoon version of "Old Joe," began appearing in U.S. advertising and promotional pieces for R.J. Reynolds.

In 1991, the *Journal of the American Medical Association* published a study showing that preschoolers recognized the Joe Camel cartoon logo as quickly as Mickey Mouse and the Disney Channel logo.

Internal documents produced in court in the case of *Mangini v. R.J. Reynolds Tobacco Company* revealed the industry's interest in targeting children as future smokers. A 1974 marketing plan stated that the "young adult market . . . represent[s] tomorrow's cigarette business. As this 14-24 age group matures, they will account for a key share of the total cigarette volume—for at least the next 25 years." A 1974 internal memo stressed that "virtually all [smokers] start by the age of 25" and "most smokers begin smoking regularly and select a usual brand at or before the age of 18."

In response to criticism, R.J. Reynolds published full-page, all-text advertisements in magazines denying the charges and stating that smoking is "an adult custom." R.J. Reynolds still denies that children were the target of their advertising and that their target market had been 25- to 49-year-old males.

In 2000, Joe Camel disappeared from all advertising and marketing pieces.

Bal remembers. It took ten months to release his department's one hundred million dollars; later, the legislature would try to cut the amount to fifty million. The Society, knowing this would cripple Bal's innovative programs, sued the state to force it to restore the money. "The Society was very supportive of me personally and of the American society," Dr. Bal commented. "The good people won out."

In 1995, California became the first state to make public and private workplaces and restaurants smoke-free. In 1998, bars were made smoke-free. California now has smoke-free schools, shopping malls, playgrounds, parks, and beaches. The California measures have made an enormous impact on smokers: California adults now purchase about forty-five packs of cigarettes per person per year—a 32.5 percent decrease since 1988. (Despite the sharp reduction, it still translates into $8.41 billion in annual smoking-related health costs to the state.)

The Society took what it learned in California and began to give support to volunteers all over the country who started grassroots efforts to ban smoking in public places. Today, more than half of all Americans live under smoke-free laws at the state or local level. The Society has also helped establish youth programs such as the Campaign for Tobacco-Free Kids, an advocacy organization that directly fights the tobacco industry's efforts to target young people. Targeting kids is a longtime trick of cigarette manufacturers. In a dramatic confession, the maker of Chesterfield cigarettes settled twenty-two state lawsuits in 1997 by admitting the industry markets cigarettes to teenagers and agreeing to warn on every pack that smoking is addictive. (Seeing the writing on the wall, R.J. Reynolds eliminated Joe Camel some time later.)

Matthew Myers, president of the Campaign for Tobacco-Free Kids, says his organization works "arm in arm" with the Society in dividing up tasks at the national level and has partnered with the Society globally in negotiating support of worldwide tobacco control efforts. Since 1997, smoking among children younger than eighteen has dropped from more than 37 percent to 22 percent, with the combined efforts of the Society and the Campaign. Smoking is at the lowest rate since the Campaign began keeping records—still unacceptably high, says Myers, but "we have made extra efforts that are the direct result of the coordination with the American Cancer Society."

The fight never ends, however, and Society leaders acknowledge it will last long past their own lifetimes; in 2006, the tobacco industry was spending twenty-eight times more than the states in their respective efforts. In 2003, the last year for which industry numbers are available, cigarette companies spent $15.2 billion on advertising and promotional expenses—more than forty-one million dollars per day.

And the tobacco industry often finds implicit partners where it shouldn't. Speaking in mid-2006, Dr. Thun pointed out Big Tobacco's new efforts to repackage smokeless tobacco (snuff) as an alternative to smoking and smoking cessation aids, with the implications that snuff is safer than other forms of tobacco. Smith Barney financial advisors were pitching the new product line to investors as a good investment.

"The show never stops," Thun says of the tobacco industry's remarkable resilience, even in the face of almost constant damnation. "It's too lucrative."

Right: Approximately three million children entered the first grade in 1988. These children were to be the high school graduates of the class of 2000, and as such were targeted as the ambassadors of a smoke-free society. A coalition of the American Cancer Society, the American Heart Association, and the American Lung Association, "Smoke-Free Class of 2000" was a tobacco education and awareness program aimed at reducing children's cigarette smoking by the end of the decade. The children pictured, shown sometime in their third-grade year, are from Decatur, Georgia.

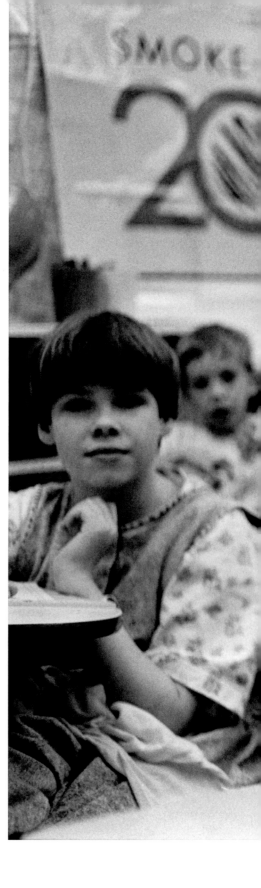

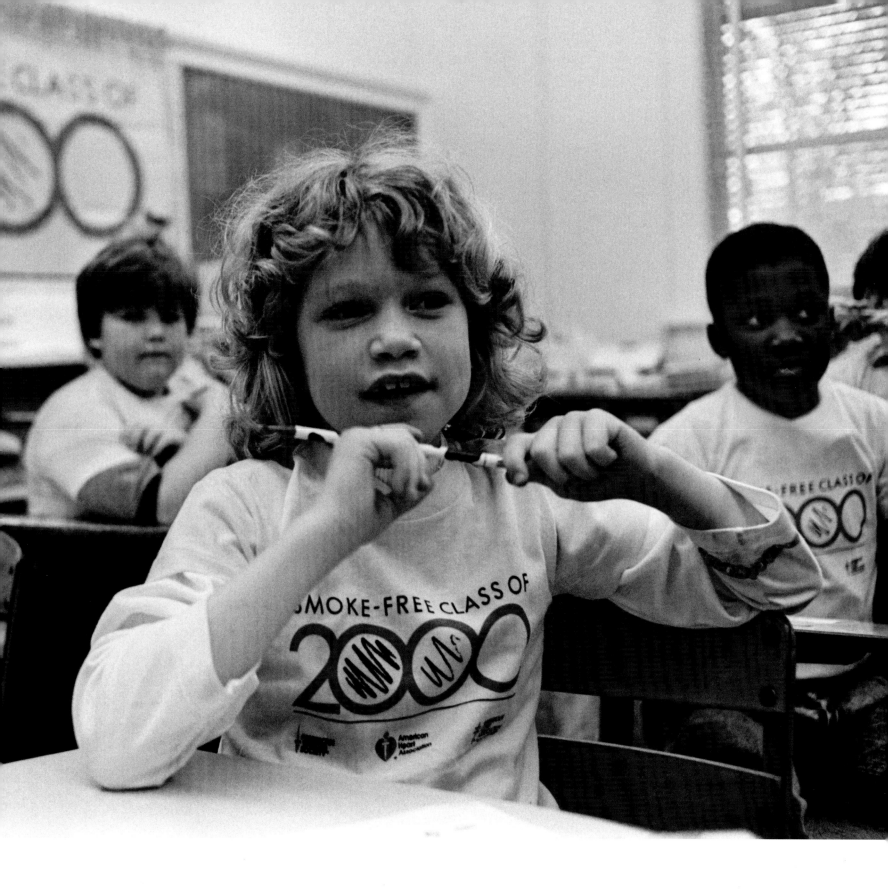

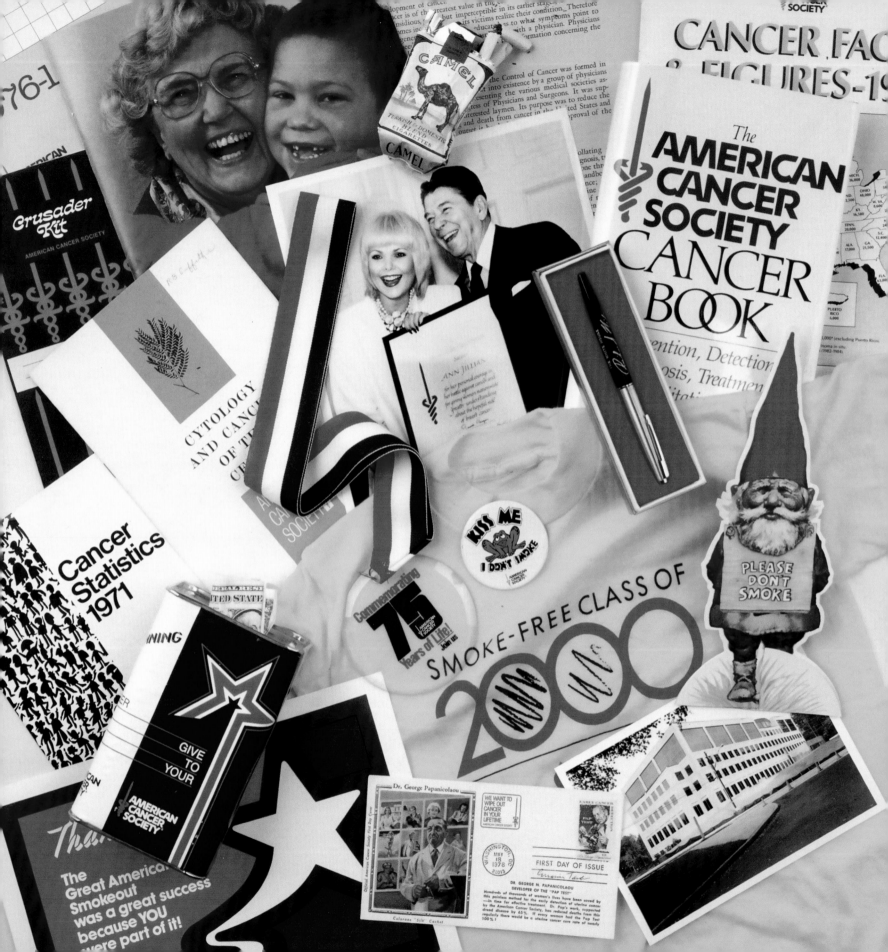

The "New" Society:
Forty Years in the Making

CHAPTER SIX

Lane Adams was the first one to see it—though not the last to try to fix it.

Fourteen years after Mary Lasker and her allies successfully brought about a major reorganization of the American Cancer Society, the troops were in revolt, the National Home Office had a weak management team, and the Society's role in seeking a cure for cancer was being fractured by in-house politics. Even though the Society was raising about thirty million dollars a year, more money than ever, its effectiveness seemed to be slipping away.

Adams, a Utah banker and Society volunteer, was hired in 1959 to be executive vice president, equivalent to today's CEO. It was a

Left: A collection of items contained in the Society's time capsule, which was sealed in 1989

job he had neither sought nor wanted; he had a wife, two children in school, and was the obvious successor to the president at a Salt Lake City bank. He was also a Utah boy, one of five brothers, used to a life of hunting, fishing, and duck shooting. He wouldn't find much of that in New York City, where the National Home Office was located.

Instead, Adams found rivalry, jealousy, distrust between the Divisions and the National Home Office, and concern from the Divisions that the 40 percent being allocated to the national budget was not being used as efficiently or effectively as it could be.

Both the strength and the weakness of the Society had always been in its strong

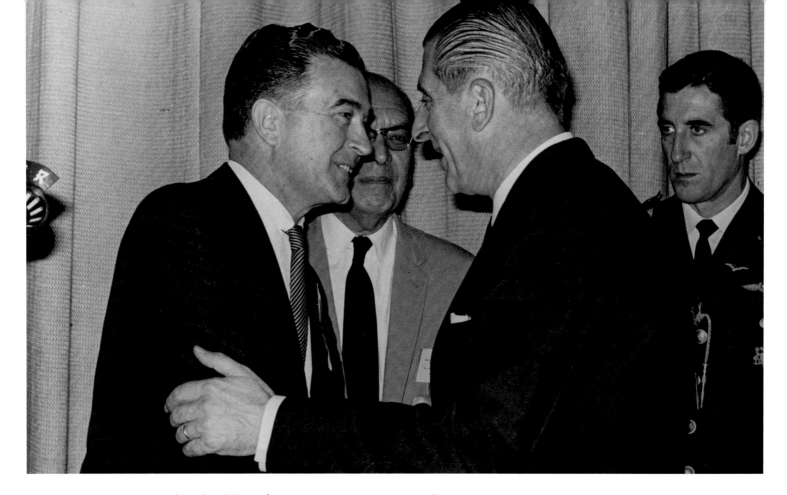

grassroots organization, and in the ability of its local Divisions to raise money for the fight against cancer. The founders of the Society, predominantly from large eastern cities, had early on recognized the need to strengthen support all over the country. They courted physicians to head state Divisions and encouraged Divisions to come up with their own programs, create their own budgets, and, in effect, run their own entities. As the Divisions grew stronger, however, their leaders (now often laypeople) looked less and less favorably on sending "their" money out of their own areas. Additionally, there were interdivisional rivalries: big states with lots of money, such as New York, were developing

innovative programs; smaller Divisions were left to create smaller, less ambitious programs. And every Division, no matter what size, felt the National Home Office was weak and inefficient, with little solid leadership.

Adams thought it would take about three years to work out the problems, and then he'd return to Salt Lake. He stayed twenty-six years. He used those years to try to unite the national headquarters and Divisions through strong nationwide programs and intense personal fundraising. He grew close to wealthy donors like Mary Lasker and her "little lambs," and he strengthened the national staff and took steps to ensure the Society was an attractive career choice. Under

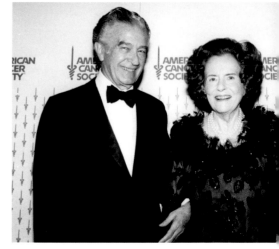

Opposite top left: Lane Adams (left) greets Eduardo Nicanor Frei Montalva, president of the Republic of Chile, at the Latin American Regional Conference on Cancer Control and related activities in 1967. Opposite bottom left: Lane Adams and Mary Lasker. It was Lasker who helped spearhead a previous reorganization of the Society. Right: Lane Adams came to the Society in 1959 to help with a much-needed reorganization. He figured he would stay for three years; he stayed for twenty-six.

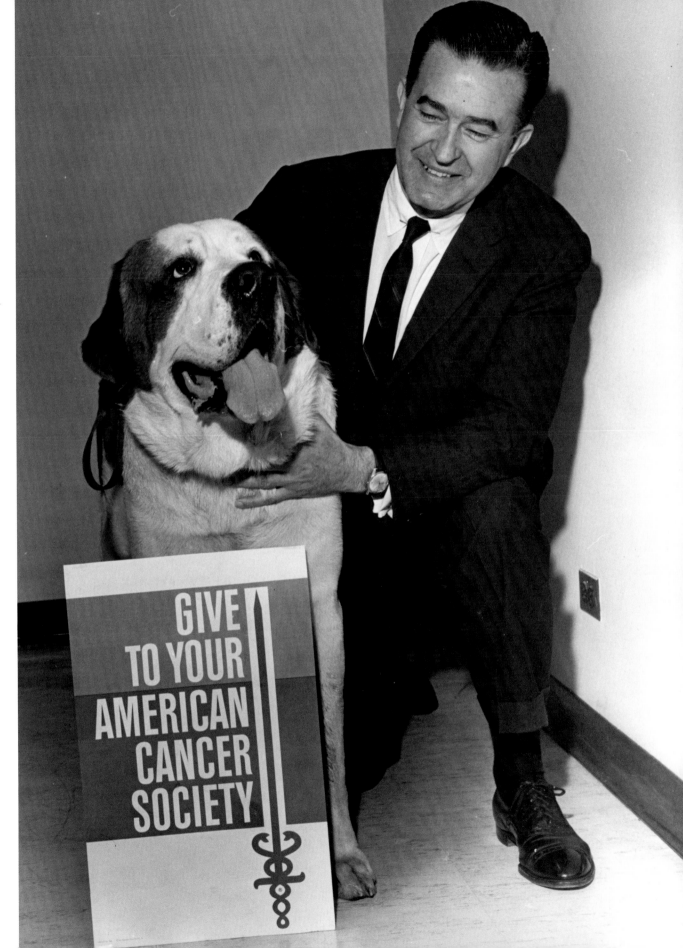

GIVE TO YOUR AMERICAN CANCER SOCIETY

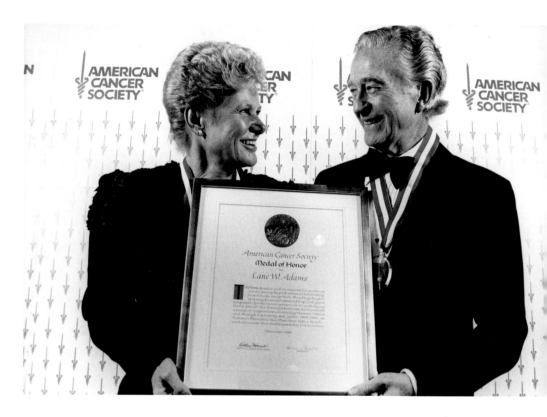

his guidance, the second Cancer Prevention Study (CPS II) was organized, and a research development program was set up to provide funds to scientists at critical junctures in their research. He helped convince the government to put more money into the National Cancer Institute—then decided the Society should never accept any of those funds, to avoid any hint of conflict of interest.

What Adams lost in good will among the Divisions—and there were those who felt no love for him—he made up in enormous leaps in nationwide programs. "It seems to me," he told Dr. Arthur Holleb, vice president for medical affairs, "that one of life's basic purposes is to be interested in the welfare of other people, and cancer is the health problem affecting most people in most ways." But while Adams's consummate skill in management and his leadership by inspiration helped the Society grow from an organization that raised twenty-eight million dollars in 1960 to one that raised two hundred fifty million in 1985, he could never entirely cure the problems he'd found his first month on the job: rivalry, jealousy, and distrust.

An Iowa Landscape

Don Thomas, the Society's chief operations officer until his retirement in 2008, wouldn't exactly have used words like "jealousy" and "distrust" to describe what was happening within the Society in the early 1990s, a few years after Adams left. Then again, he was working in the Florida Division, a successful

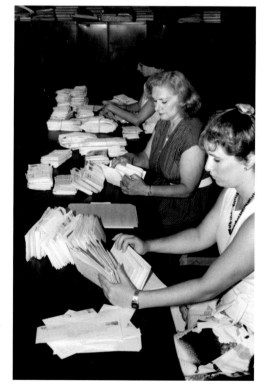

Division funding huge numbers of patient service and cancer prevention programs. He had an enviable position as executive vice president, one he'd earned from twenty-five years as part of an organization he loved. When he thought about it, he'd had a good run.

Thomas was a senior at the University of Florida in 1968 majoring in public relations when the Society came on his screen—literally. One of his senior assignments was to do a public relations campaign for a non-profit organization. The U.S. government had ordered television stations to allow free anti-tobacco spots as part of the Fairness Doctrine it adopted as more and more negative reports emerged about smoking. The government recognized that the tobacco industry had millions and millions to spend on promoting

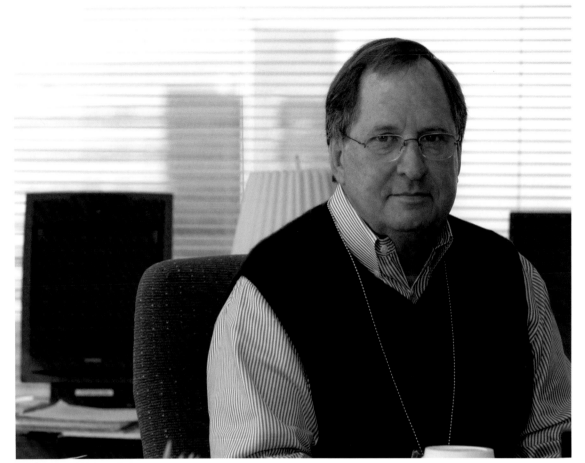

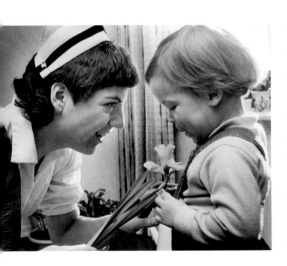

Opposite top: Kathleen J. Horsch and Lane Adams. Adams was awarded the Society's Medal of Honor in 1988 for his outstanding leadership and achievements. Opposite bottom: Workers sort surveys as part of Cancer Prevention Study II. Right: Don Thomas's association with the Society began as a college assignment. From there, he went to work in a local Florida office of the Society and by the time he retired in 2008—forty years later—he had risen to the highest echelons of the organization. Below: Susan Skiles, RN, hands young Jeremy Reinhold a daffodil in 1982. Daffodil Days® is one of the American Cancer Society's oldest and most beloved fundraisers.

their products, but anti-tobacco groups were cash strapped. One of the Society's spots came on the television while Thomas was deciding which nonprofit to choose. Figuring the American Cancer Society was "a good organization," Thomas went to the local office in Gainesville and was referred first to the regional office in Atlanta, then to the National Home Office in New York City.

By the time Thomas completed his senior year, he'd been offered a job by the Society in the Florida Division as a national trainee, assigned to organize a door-to-door residential crusade in Orange County, Florida, with a goal of raising thirty-five thousand dollars. Eventually, he became

director of field operations in fundraising in the Florida Division, then deputy executive vice president, and then executive vice president. It was a straight shot up.

Lane Adams had retired in 1985, and there had been a seven-year struggle to find the right person to replace him. The gap exacerbated some of the problems Adams had identified as far back as 1959. In many ways, the problems came with growth—under Adams's leadership, the Society expanded to fifty-eight Divisions, more than thirty-two hundred local affiliate offices, and 2.5 million volunteers. There were some two hundred national committees, subcommittees, task forces, and other working groups reporting to the National Board of Directors—which itself had 220 members who met three times a year. There were also about thirty-six hundred staff members nationwide—eighteen hundred who managed the other eighteen hundred, Thomas thought.

While the growth was good in one sense, it also created a more sprawling, harder-to-manage organization. The organizational chart, recalls Gary J. Streit, an Iowa lawyer and volunteer who later became chair of the board in 2004, "looked like an Iowa landscape with all the silos."

In addition, the Society had made a controversial decision to move its National Home Office out of New York City and to Atlanta in 1989, turning the entire organization upside down. The Society had spent its first seventy-five years headquartered in New York, where people "thought the world ended at the Hudson River," laughs Dr. John Lazlo, who was then national vice president for research. The logistics of the move were no laughing matter, however. Less than 25 percent of the national staff chose to relocate to Atlanta, a percentage consultants had predicted. Many who did choose to move were initially doing the work of two or three people, including building a computer system from scratch.

Three cities were the finalists for the chance to host the Society headquarters, and it was a difficult decision. Eventually, however,

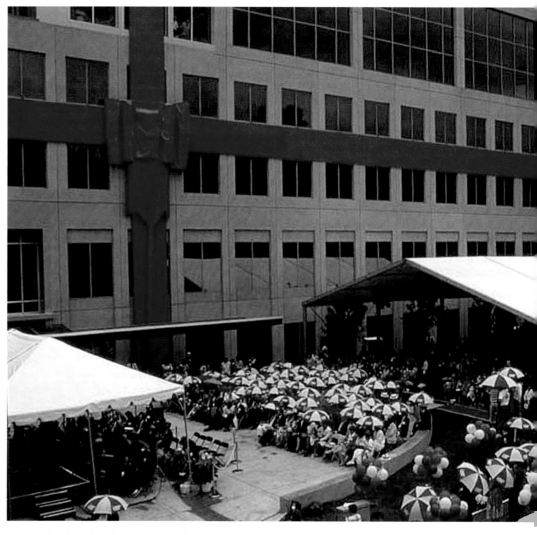

Society leaders decided that one of the top reasons to move was the opportunity to partner with Emory University and the Centers for Disease Control, both right across the street.

The move, coupled with the arrival of the third chief executive officer in seven years, had by the early 1990s left the Divisions no happier with national than they had been when Adams first arrived. In 1993, leaders of the larger Divisions sat down for a meeting in California to launch a campaign to reduce

Above: Dedication of the then-new National Home Office headquarters in Georgia. Attracted by the nearby U.S. Centers for Disease Control and Emory University, the Society made a controversial decision to relocate to Atlanta in 1989. The organization had spent seventy-five years in New York City. Opposite: Dr. John Seffrin came to the Society in 1992 as chief executive officer and began the difficult process of rerouting the massive ship that the organization had become.

to the National Board of Directors—which itself had 220 members who met three times a year. There were also about thirty-six hundred staff members nationwide—eighteen hundred who managed the other eighteen hundred, Thomas thought.

While the growth was good in one sense, it also created a more sprawling, harder-to-manage organization. The organizational chart, recalls Gary J. Streit, an Iowa lawyer and volunteer who later became chair of the board in 2004, "looked like an Iowa landscape with all the silos."

In addition, the Society had made a controversial decision to move its National Home Office out of New York City and to Atlanta in 1989, turning the entire organization upside down. The Society had spent its first seventy-five years headquartered in New York, where people "thought the world ended at the Hudson River," laughs Dr. John Lazlo, who was then national vice president for research. The logistics of the move were no laughing matter, however. Less than 25 percent of the national staff chose to relocate to Atlanta, a percentage consultants had predicted. Many who did choose to move were initially doing the work of two or three people, including building a computer system from scratch.

Three cities were the finalists for the chance to host the Society headquarters, and it was a difficult decision. Eventually, however,

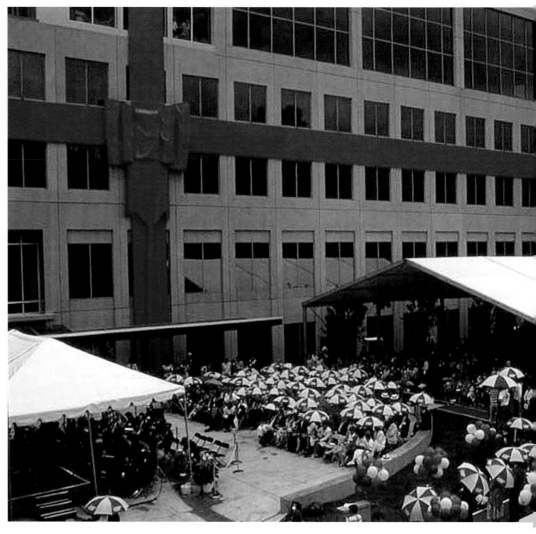

Society leaders decided that one of the top reasons to move was the opportunity to partner with Emory University and the Centers for Disease Control, both right across the street.

The move, coupled with the arrival of the third chief executive officer in seven years, had by the early 1990s left the Divisions no happier with national than they had been when Adams first arrived. In 1993, leaders of the larger Divisions sat down for a meeting in California to launch a campaign to reduce

Above: Dedication of the then-new National Home Office headquarters in Georgia. Attracted by the nearby U.S. Centers for Disease Control and Emory University, the Society made a controversial decision to relocate to Atlanta in 1989. The organization had spent seventy-five years in New York City. Opposite: Dr. John Seffrin came to the Society in 1992 as chief executive officer and began the difficult process of rerouting the massive ship that the organization had become.

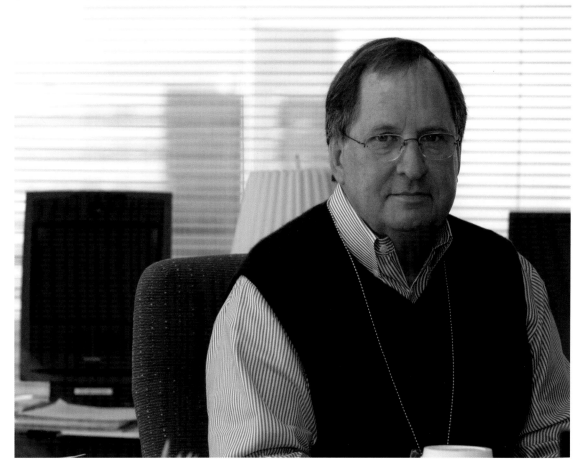

Opposite top: Kathleen J. Horsch and Lane Adams. Adams was awarded the Society's Medal of Honor in 1988 for his outstanding leadership and achievements. Opposite bottom: Workers sort surveys as part of Cancer Prevention Study II. Right: Don Thomas's association with the Society began as a college assignment. From there, he went to work in a local Florida office of the Society and by the time he retired in 2008—forty years later—he had risen to the highest echelons of the organization. Below: Susan Skiles, RN, hands young Jeremy Reinhold a daffodil in 1982. Daffodil Days® is one of the American Cancer Society's oldest and most beloved fundraisers.

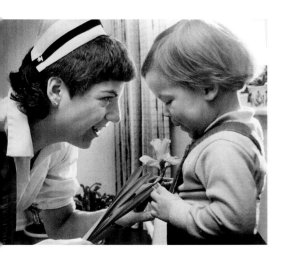

their products, but anti-tobacco groups were cash strapped. One of the Society's spots came on the television while Thomas was deciding which nonprofit to choose. Figuring the American Cancer Society was "a good organization," Thomas went to the local office in Gainesville and was referred first to the regional office in Atlanta, then to the National Home Office in New York City.

By the time Thomas completed his senior year, he'd been offered a job by the Society in the Florida Division as a national trainee, assigned to organize a door-to-door residential crusade in Orange County, Florida, with a goal of raising thirty-five thousand dollars. Eventually, he became director of field operations in fundraising in the Florida Division, then deputy executive vice president, and then executive vice president. It was a straight shot up.

Lane Adams had retired in 1985, and there had been a seven-year struggle to find the right person to replace him. The gap exacerbated some of the problems Adams had identified as far back as 1959. In many ways, the problems came with growth—under Adams's leadership, the Society expanded to fifty-eight Divisions, more than thirty-two hundred local affiliate offices, and 2.5 million volunteers. There were some two hundred national committees, subcommittees, task forces, and other working groups reporting

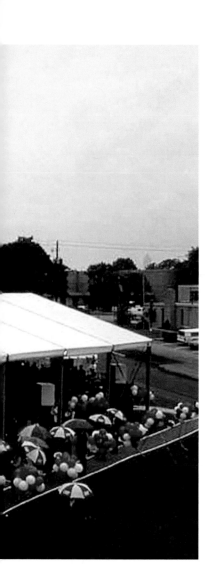

the percentage sent to the National Home Office from 40 percent to 20 percent. Such talk was heresy: the 60-40 split was a sacred cow. For them to even think of this change showed the deep distrust and unhappiness they felt for the Society's national leadership.

Yet the National Home Office had its own reason to be unhappy: from 1988 to 1992, donations to the Society had stagnated, barely increasing 1 or 2 percent a year, and some of the Divisions were struggling just to raise enough money to pay salaries. "When it gets down to really delivering programs," one Division executive told Thomas, "we're not."

Welcoming the Enemy

Not all of this was news to Dr. John Seffrin, who had been chair of the board in 1990 before he was hired in 1992 to be chief executive officer, though he hadn't realized the depths of the problem until he became CEO. All the issues that Thomas and the other Division executives talked about were the same things with which Seffrin was struggling. Working like a madman—giving up nights and weekends, scheduling himself to endless travel around the Divisions—Seffrin was slowly, slowly pulling the Society back together. He was warm, congenial, "a real gentleman," as one volunteer described him, and he really listened to the Division leadership concerns.

Yet he had very set ideas about what he wanted the Society to represent, including a stronger role in the public health arena, a higher profile internationally, and an

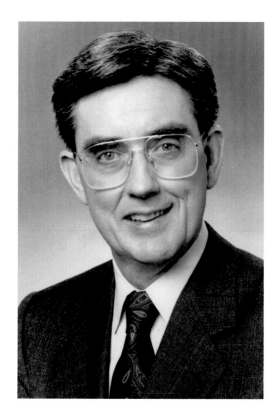

improved educational resource for cancer patients. He needed the goodwill of the Division leadership to do that. But meeting every other month with the Division CEOs and the senior staff was "more like a convention," says Seffrin. "It was not a meeting in the normal sense of the word."

Seffrin knew he could not accomplish his long-range goals until he solved the organizational and fundraising dilemmas.

What Dr. Seffrin was seeking—much like the Divisions—was leadership, someone who could help solve the day-to-day problems and let him get on with the outreach he felt was necessary for the Society's future. Seffrin recognized the answers probably lay with someone

in the field who was familiar with the problems and ready to help solve them. Who better than the Florida Division's Don Thomas, who had been the only other finalist for the job of CEO when the Society hired Seffrin?

Seffrin had already worked with Thomas during the crisis over the Divisions' request to lower the percentage they sent to national. Thomas had carried the message from the California meeting to Chairman of the Board Stanley Shmishkiss, a real estate and insurance businessman from Massachusetts. Thomas had first briefed Seffrin, then in his early months as CEO, about what the Divisions wanted. Together, with the support of the board, they'd worked out a compromise.

Thomas, who retired in 2008 after forty years with the Society, admits that the staff of the national headquarters groaned when Seffrin announced he had been hired as deputy executive vice president for field operations. "It sent shock waves through the organization, because I was the absolute worst critic of national. And all of a sudden, now I'm one of them. I'd gone over from the 'we' to the 'they.'"

The Society was poised for its next major reorganization. Not only was it too sprawling an organization to manage effectively, but a tremendous and expensive duplication of services was also taking place within Divisions, draining off energy and resources that could be better used to fight cancer.

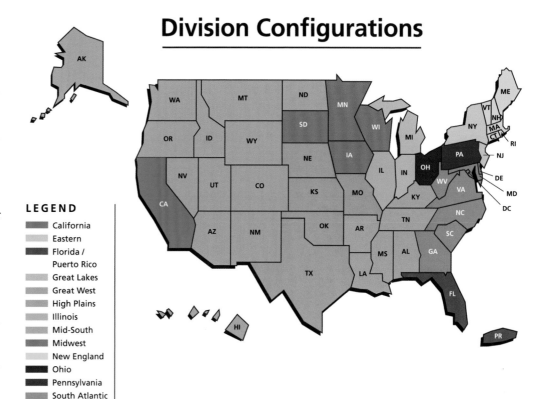

Division Configurations

LEGEND
- California
- Eastern
- Florida / Puerto Rico
- Great Lakes
- Great West
- High Plains
- Illinois
- Mid-South
- Midwest
- New England
- Ohio
- Pennsylvania
- South Atlantic

Such a reorganization was complicated both politically and legally; each one of the Divisions was a separate corporation that would have to be dissolved, then new Divisions legally re-formed. Francis L. Coolidge, a Boston attorney and a member of the board's bylaws committee, took on the job of helping to guide the Society through the process.

Helped in great part by the legal terms set down by Coolidge, the Society began the drastic restructuring. Pivotal was a reduction in the number of Divisions and a consolidation of services. National and Division leadership began to move around the country, sharing the concept of reorgan-

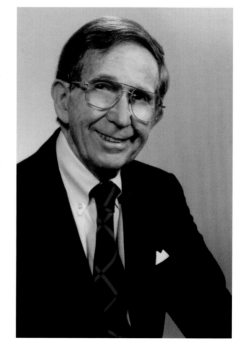

ization with volunteers and staff angry and hurt at the idea of giving up the programs and organization they had nurtured for so many years. There were times, Seffrin and Thomas admit, when they weren't sure they were going to get out of town alive. At one meeting of a Divisional executive committee, a woman volunteer sitting across the table clearly wanted to leap across the table and strangle Thomas. In another instance, Thomas traveled to a major city to meet with the volunteer president of one Division who had demanded a face-to-face meeting. She picked him up at the train station on a cold, rainy day and took him to a little coffee shop. With admiration, Thomas says, "I didn't know there was a woman who could swear as much as that woman swore."

After 1996, the fifty-eight Division offices were consolidated into thirteen geographic Divisions, and the national board went from two hundred twenty to forty-three members. Divisional staffing costs dropped, and more money became available to develop programs to help prevent cancer and serve cancer survivors—always the real passion of the volunteers. Two-thirds of the way through the reorganization, the Society was saving up to thirty million dollars a year in redundant costs. Gradually, the National Home Office also began to manage centrally some of the tasks the Divisions had done, such as paying bills and warehousing materials, allowing even more cost savings.

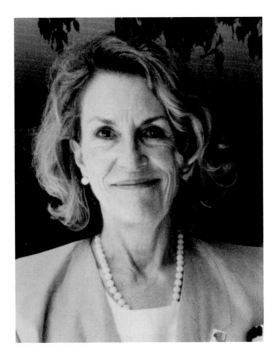

There were some downsides to the mergers. A number of board members who had had significant roles were displaced, and some felt the mergers had diminished the Society's commitment to volunteers. In retrospect, Seffrin said he should have spent at least as much time focusing on volunteers as he did taking care of staff, and he should have had a more proactive plan to deal with disaffected volunteers. "We're still dealing with that—thankfully to a lesser extent," he acknowledged in 2007.

Triple Five

Even before the reorganization, Seffrin had begun to take steps to try to solve the flat revenue problems. Seffrin had agreed with Thomas that day in 1992 when he presented numbers showing that the Divisions bore

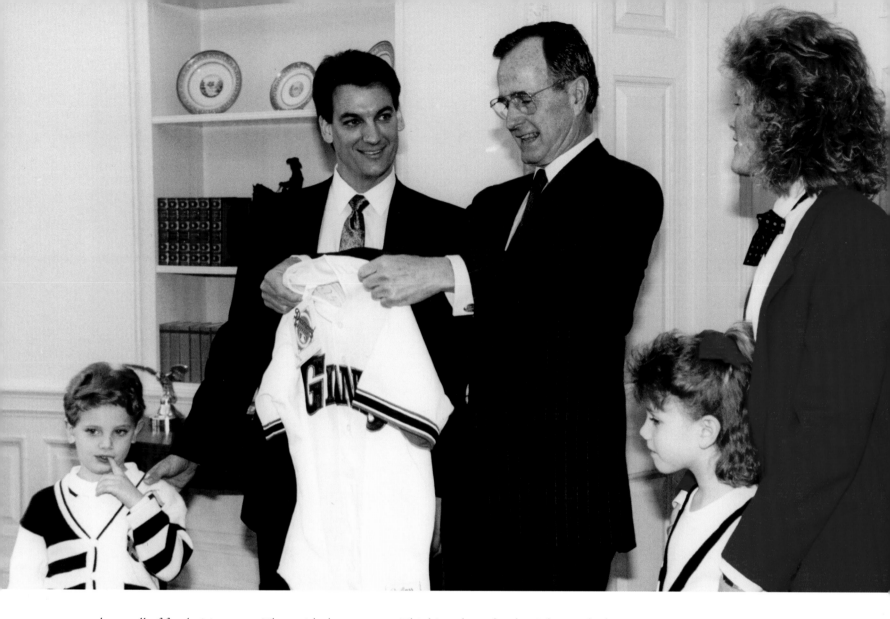

almost all of fundraising costs. That, with the 40 percent that was going back to national, left the Divisions with less and less to spend locally on fighting cancer and serving patients. If the board wouldn't agree to lower the 40 percent split, would they agree to pick up some of those costs? When Shmishkiss asked his opinion, Seffrin spoke carefully. Don had made his case, he said, and I think we "have to do something here."

Thinking through what Thomas had said, Seffrin proposed what would become known as the "Triple Five Program." National would return an additional 5 percent of fundraising income each year for three years, beginning in 1993, to Divisions. That additional income would be used specifically to recruit volunteers and to develop the infrastructure for improving fundraising. Seffrin believed the money

Above: Former San Francisco Giants pitcher Dave Dravecky and his family share a moment with President George H. W. Bush. Dravecky was awarded the American Cancer Society Courage Award by President Bush in 1990. Opposite: While president of the Society in 1994, Dr. Irvin Fleming, a renowned oncologist, made the difficult decision to cut some of the research funding to help the organization through a difficult period.

Cancer Milestones in the 1990s

1990s—The American Cancer Society advocates for cancer prevention and quality of life for cancer survivors by working to pass the Nutrition Labeling and Education Act, the Breast and Cervical Cancer Mortality Prevention Act, Medicare coverage of mammograms and other cancer screening exams, the Americans with Disabilities Act, the Mammography Quality Standards Act, the Family and Medical Leave Act, and the Health Insurance Portability and Accountability Act.

1990—Mary-Claire King, PhD, discovers a breast cancer gene, demonstrating that breast cancer can be inherited.

1991—American Cancer Society–funded research shows young children recognize Joe Camel as easily as Mickey Mouse.

1992—The American Cancer Society Foundation holds its first Board of Trustees meeting. Founding trustees are Stanley Shmishkiss, David Bethune, Gordon Binder, Mrs. Elmer H. Bobst, Ralph Destino, William J. Flynn, Walter Lawrence, MD, Senator Connie Mack III, Howard Marguleas, and Diane Disney Miller.

1993—The first American Cancer Society's Making Strides Against Breast Cancer® is held in Boston.

1994—The American Cancer Society's Man to Man® program begins, offering support and information for men with prostate cancer.

1995—With support to the American Cancer Society Foundation from the Leo and Gloria Rosen family, the American Cancer Society's Web site, www.cancer.org, is launched.

1995—With early support from the American Cancer Society Foundation and the vision of volunteer Lana Rosenfeld, "tlc" Tender Loving Care®, is published. The Society's "magalog" provides cancer patients and survivors with innovative products and apparel at low cost.

1997—The American Cancer Society dedicates the majority of its research dollars to beginning investigators.

1997—The Society's toll-free number, 800-227-2345, is launched, eventually providing information 24 hours a day, 7 days a week.

1997—The American Cancer Society, the Centers for Disease Control and Prevention, and the National Cancer Institute jointly announce the first documented overall downturn in cancer mortality: overall cancer death rates fall 0.5 percent per year between 1991 and 1995.

1997—The FDA approves monoclonal antibody therapy for lymphoma, based on the work of Society Clinical Research Professor Ronald Levy, MD.

1998—The Society announces that the number of people being diagnosed with cancer decreases for the first time.

1998—Former Society grantee Dennis Slamon, MD, shows that a genetically engineered, "humanized" monoclonal antibody, Herceptin, improves survival of women with advanced breast cancer.

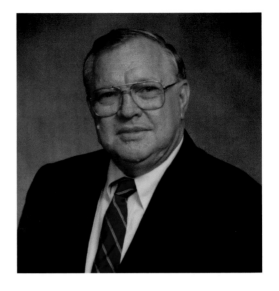

would increase the annual fundraising enough to offset Triple Five—a gamble some others at the Society thought was crazy.

The National Home Office would have to cut its budget 5 percent each year to make the return. Thomas, hired within the first year of Triple Five, suddenly found himself on the other end of the stick, trying to cut his own budget to feed the Divisions. The first 5 percent came pretty easily; the next year, Thomas had to squeeze harder to get the money.

The research budget at the Society had always been sacrosanct; cancer research was the reason many donors gave, believing that if anyone could find a cure for cancer, it would be the Society. Yet it became obvious in the second year of Triple Five that the Research department was also going to have to bear some of the brunt of budget trimming. Seffrin arranged a meeting at the Atlanta airport with Dr. Irvin Fleming, then president, and Larry Fuller, chair of the

board, to break the news. The spreadsheet Seffrin carried told the story in a way he couldn't: Without the cuts, the Society was going to be one hundred million dollars in debt in eight to ten years. With the cuts, the Society could sustain the Triple Five program—which Seffrin's other spreadsheet showed was starting to work by increasing donations—indefinitely.

It was a tough decision, one of those an organization sometimes has to make to survive. "I've always given great credit to Irv," says Seffrin. "He was a doctor, and a famous one, and doctors are generally the biggest supporters of research. But he said, 'Do it.'"

By the third year, the new Divisions had dug themselves out of their financial hole. Donations began to rise, and faith in the national leadership was going up even faster. Instead of sending the cash back to the Divisions, the board decided to put that year's 5 percent into a general pool to start something everyone thought would be an asset to the Society and the public: a twenty-four-hour national call center for cancer information (see Chapter 8, "The Warm Hand of Service").

Lucky Breaks and Hard-Earned Results

While board chair in 1990, Seffrin had asked Dr. Harmon Eyre, the Society's president in 1988, to come back again as a volunteer to head a committee to define the Society's priorities for the 1990s. It was the first real attempt as an organization to prioritize the work the Society did based on its mission, and it illustrated Seffrin's desire to set the Society on a path that would carry it forward for years, no matter its leadership. Ultimately, Eyre and his committee produced Mission 2000, a strategic plan to close the gap between the existing burden of cancer deaths and disability and the goals implicit in the Society's mission statement. Internal and external factors drove Mission 2000. The primary external factor was increasing competition for money, time, volunteers, and most important, public attention. Internal factors included the increasingly vocal message from the Divisions that they were stretched too thin with too few resources.

Mission 2000 was the first step toward refocusing the Society's efforts on the essential strategies that would help it accomplish its mission, but leaders felt more was needed. National leaders and the board began work on a plan to focus the Society's work for the most impact. With the support of David Zacks (who would later serve as board chair in 2003), the plan of work developed into five strategic directions. These goals were an affirmation of the tenets that had been an essential part of the Society for so long: delivery of quality information, collaboration with others, commitment to research, advocacy for others, and financial responsibility. The strategic directions helped refocus the Society's energies and, in time, would help turn the Society's work into tangible results.

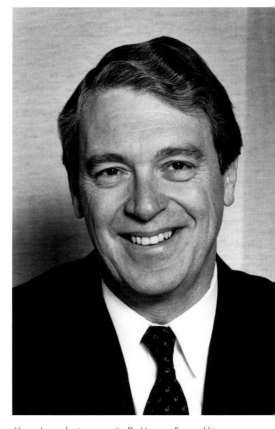

Above: In a volunteer capacity, Dr. Harmon Eyre and his committee produced Mission 2000, a blueprint to close the gap between the reality of cancer and the Society's mission statement. He came on staff in 1993 as chief medical officer. Opposite: The January/February 1997 issue of *CA: A Cancer Journal for Clinicians*, with the headline "First Decline in Overall Cancer Mortality"

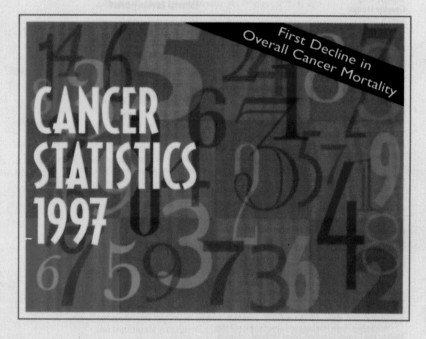

CA

January / February 1997
Vol. 47 No. 1

A CANCER JOURNAL FOR CLINICIANS

First Decline in Overall Cancer Mortality

CANCER STATISTICS 1997

ALSO IN THIS ISSUE

**TUMOR-RELATED PROGNOSTIC FACTORS IN BREAST CANCER
PATHOBIOLOGICAL CONSIDERATIONS IN DCIS**

American Cancer Society, Inc.
1599 Clifton Road, N.E.
Atlanta, Georgia 30329

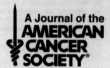

A Journal of the
AMERICAN CANCER SOCIETY®

1-800-ACS-2345
http://www.cancer.org

Non-Profit Org.
U.S.POSTAGE
PAID
Permit No. 2203
Nashville, TN

Seffrin again turned to Eyre in 1993, asking him to join the staff to oversee all the research and medical aspects of the organization as chief medical officer and executive vice president for research and cancer control science. With Thomas now running the day-to-day operations, and Eyre organizing and focusing the medical efforts to address the disease, the Society was clearly set to make the biggest impact on cancer in the new millennium. The three men also moved the Society into the international arena, with Seffrin becoming involved with the International Union Against Cancer (UICC) and Eyre overseeing international outreach.

The Society's hard-earned results are savored not just by the Society, but also by the world. November 14, 1996, became one of the most significant dates in organizational history, when the Society announced the first-ever decline in the cancer death rate in the United States. The drop was a turning point from the steady increase throughout much of the century. Although the death rate had only fallen 3 percent, based on deaths between 1991 and 1995, it marked a measurable turning of the tide against cancer. For the Society, however, it was only the beginning. That year, the Society declared its commitment to accelerate this decline and to achieve a 50 percent reduction in cancer deaths by 2015 (see Chapter 10, "2015 and Beyond"). There would be more milestones, and much more work to come.

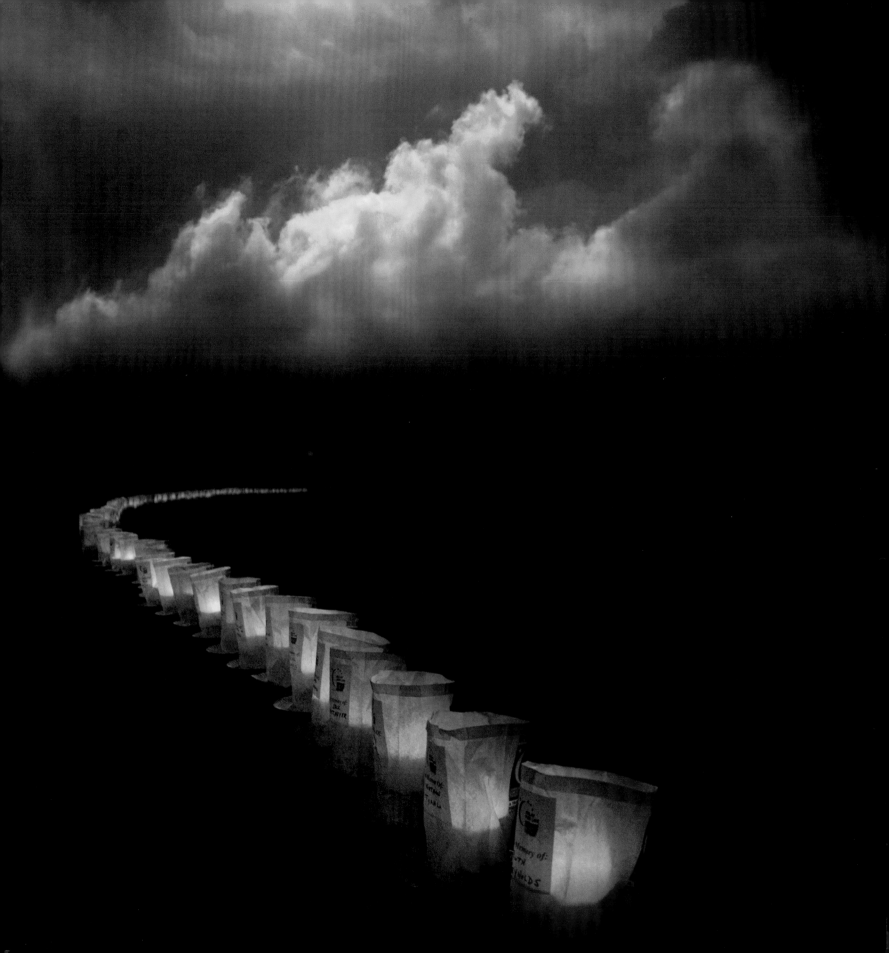

Victory Laps

The sound of the bagpipes playing "Amazing Grace" is haunting. It hangs in the damp, spring air of the island of Martha's Vineyard, Massachusetts, the mournful tune contrasting sharply with the unsung words: "Amazing grace, how sweet the sound, that saved a wretch like me . . ." Following behind the piper on the track are a few hundred walkers—some moving slowly, some chatting quietly with friends, all reminded by the piping of why they are there, of who they want to remember—and how. "Through many dangers, toils and snares, we have already come."

The luminaria are lit, and the names carefully written on their sides, lovingly decorated with stars and roses and rainbows. Each name has a story—sometimes of pain, sometimes of hope and healing. Some of the people whose names are on the bags have earlier circled the track in the traditional Survivors Lap, an emotional, cathartic trip that left eyes brimming and a few hands pumped into the air with the sign of victory.

The American Cancer Society Relay For Life® on Martha's Vineyard only began in 2004, and it is held in a community of just

Opposite: At a Relay For Life event, luminaria with names written on the sides give testimony to stories of life, hope, memory, and healing. The Luminary Ceremony is one part of Relay For Life, which enables participants to celebrate, remember, and fight back against cancer.

fifteen thousand people. Although the Vineyard is known as an exclusive vacation resort for the wealthy, the island's full-time residents are not wealthy, and they need every dollar just to meet a cost of living that is one-third higher than on the mainland seven miles away. Even so, the locals are very charitable; two hundred non-profits are represented on this small island, and charitable events are a part of everyday life. In that spirit, the 2006 Vineyard Relay For Life raised seventy-three thousand dollars for the American Cancer Society. "You're not going to find a cure for cancer on Martha's Vineyard," says Eleanor Beth, a two-time breast cancer survivor and one of the original organizers of the Martha's Vineyard Relay. "But those of us who knew Relays knew what donations could do and how much they can mean in the fight against cancer—and how much the Relay itself could mean to us. It's a survivor's event. It means we're fighting back."

Communities have shown this kind of dedication since 1985, when a surgeon in Tacoma, Washington, began his own one-man, twenty-four-hour fundraiser for the American Cancer Society. Since then, Relay has contributed three billion dollars to the fight against cancer and has become the Society's signature activity. Almost five thousand Relays take place annually, in all fifty

Reuel Johnson

states. Hundreds of colleges hold Relays. The smallest Relay may only raise a few thousand dollars; the largest, in Gwinnett County, Georgia, outside Atlanta, raised more than two and a half million dollars in 2007. "The growth pattern has been unprecedented," says Reuel Johnson, the Society's national vice president, Relay For Life. "It has allowed us to regain our core competency as a community-based, volunteer organization."

Johnson wasn't always a true believer. The idea of a Relay For Life gained acceptance in many communities before the national organization embraced it. "I thought it sounded a little crazy," Johnson admits. "It was hard enough getting people to spend a couple of hours doing something; how were you going to get them to spend all night?"

Something Special
Pat Flynn certainly had no plans to spend the night at the university track that windy, rainy May evening in 1985. She had heard about the twenty-four-hour run/walk a local doctor was planning, and had even pledged ten dollars. Around eleven o'clock Friday night, she'd driven the four minutes from her house to Baker Field at the University of Puget Sound in north Tacoma, peering over the fence to see what was happening. As she remembers, it was something to see.

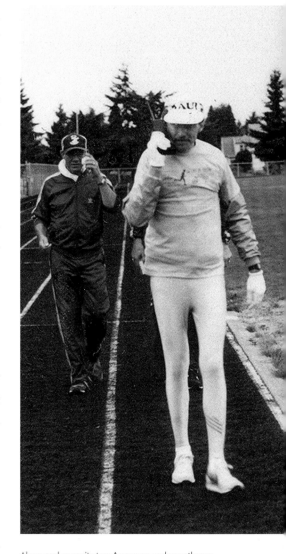

Above and opposite top: A surgeon and marathoner from Tacoma, Washington, Dr. Gordon Klatt started what would eventually become the American Cancer Society Relay For Life. In the first relay event, he was the only participant and ran and walked for twenty-four hours. Above left: Reuel Johnson, national vice president for Relay For Life for the Society, initially thought "it sounded a little crazy." He soon changed his mind. Opposite bottom right: Supporters join Dr. Gordon Klatt as he circles the track at night during the first twenty-four-hour run/walk.

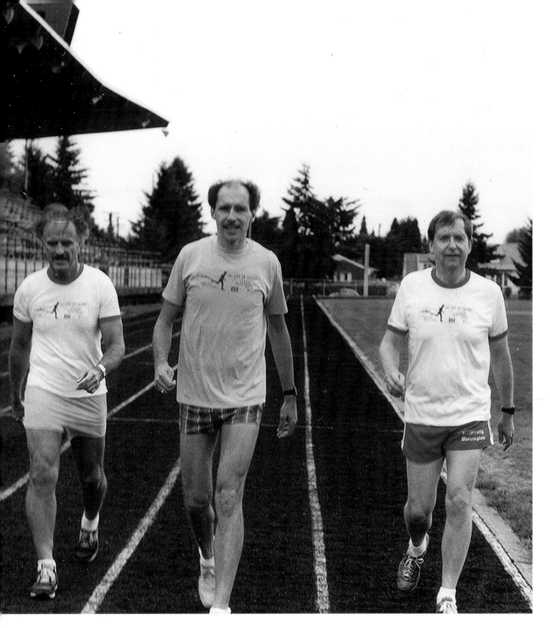

a number of years and had done public education outreach for much of that time, talking about cancer, diet, regular checkups—all the things people needed to know about colorectal cancer. When he became president, he realized he should get involved in fundraising and decided to tie his running to the cause.

Klatt knew he needed something eye-catching. What better than to say he'd stay out on that track for twenty-four hours, an entire day? He would run one lap and walk the next, with a five-minute break every hour. He trained vigorously for a year and enlisted a friend who was a cardiologist and another who was a nutritionist to be at the track. About three hundred people came out to watch him, many of them cancer patients whom he had treated. His father, who had

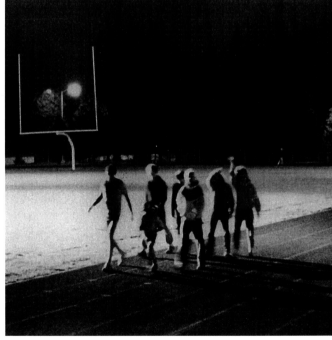

Dr. Gordon "Gordy" Klatt, a Tacoma colorectal surgeon, was on the track, sometimes alone and sometimes with people who had pledged twenty-five dollars to spend a half hour walking or running with him. Dr. Klatt, a marathon runner, had the brainstorm for this fundraiser a year earlier, when he was volunteer president of his county's Society chapter. He'd been on the local board of directors for

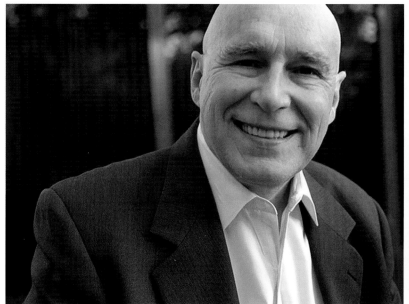

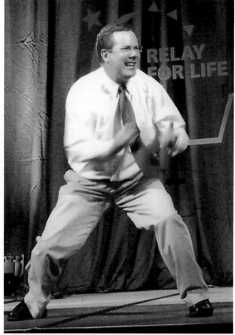

Far left: Dr. "Gordy" Klatt. Left: "Dr. Bob." Bottom left: Pat Flynn went to the track in the middle of the night to watch her physician—Dr. Klatt—making his loops, and called the newspaper to tell them to send a photographer. She was later asked to help organize Relay on a national basis. Bottom: Dr. Bob's support team

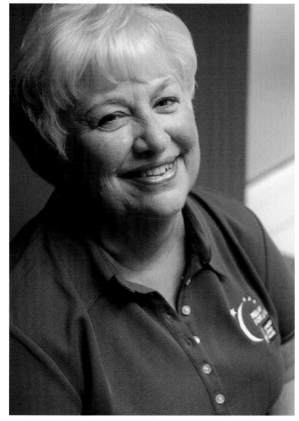

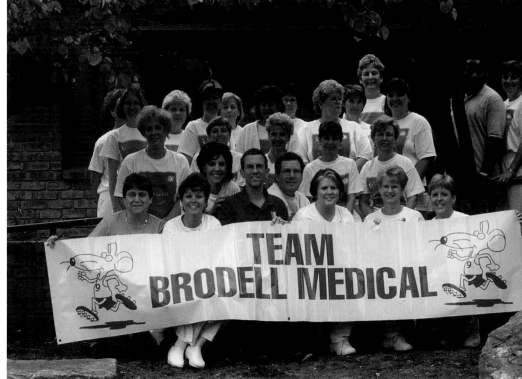

had coronary bypass surgery and was in his seventies, was at the track for hours with him.

Even with his training, his body began to rebel after ten hours, when he became hypothermic about daybreak. His blood pressure dropped, and his cardiologist had sodium-rich chicken soup waiting for him, to warm him up and replace the salt he was losing. At eighteen hours, he had to quit running and started walking. At twenty-four hours, he had walked eighty-three miles and raised twenty-seven thousand dollars for the Society.

Pat Flynn spent only a short time at the track, then went home to her husband and her bed. Around 1 a.m., she got up, dressed, and went back. She got up at 6 a.m. and went back again. She knew Dr. Klatt as her physician, but she couldn't explain what kept drawing her to the track to watch. "I just felt it was something special." In the middle of the night, she called the *Tacoma News Tribune* to tell them of the incredible effort taking place at Baker Field. They sent a photographer at six in the morning.

Dr. Klatt, exhausted but exhilarated, thought this had been something special, too. His cancer patients kept coming up to him, telling him what an inspiration the event had been to them. The doctor realized

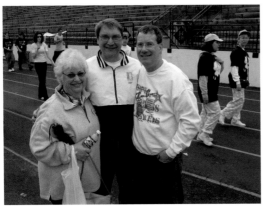

Pat Flynn, Reuel Johnson, and "Dr. Bob"

he wanted to capture that inspiration and make it a part of his life; at the same time, he knew he didn't want to run twenty-four hours every year. Someone mentioned Pat Flynn to him, telling him she'd been at the track. Flynn was involved with many community activities and was well known in Tacoma. She was also an assistant public information officer with the Tacoma School District, working with the media on a daily basis, and Klatt realized he needed someone who knew how to get publicity.

He called her a few months after the run. He needed a little help getting a committee to organize a team relay run and walk next year. Was she game?

Vision and Details

Eight years later and hundreds of miles away, Dr. Robert Brodell was pretty sure he had the answer to all of the Society's financial concerns: three-on-three basketball. It was fun, it was popular, and in his mind, it was the way to bring in valuable and needed donations.

"Dr. Bob" was a Society legacy. His father had been the president and crusade chairman for the local Society chapter in Warren, Ohio, in the days when the door-to-door campaign was the most successful and productive

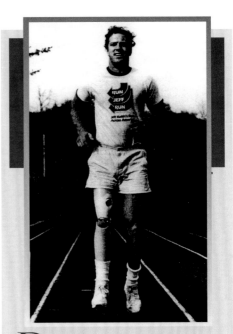

Dr. Gordon Klatt was not the first person to consider running as a way to raise money for cancer. Jeff Keith lost his leg to cancer when he was twelve years old. In 1984 he decided to run from Boston to Los Angeles to raise funds for the American Cancer Society and the National Handicapped Sports and Recreation Foundation. He left Boston on June 4, 1984, and when he arrived in Los Angeles on February 18, 1985, he became the first and only amputee to run across America. Most important, he raised more than two million dollars.

In 1992, Jeff and his friend Matt Vossler formed the nonprofit Swim Across America. Every year all across the country, they organize swim events to raise money for cancer research, treatment, and prevention. The swim events range in length from one-half mile to twenty-two miles, and they have raised more than twenty million dollars for the fight against cancer.

fundraising effort in the country. One of Dr. Bob's earliest memories was of going to Cleveland with his dad to a Society state conference and meeting Lorne Greene, the silver-haired Pa Cartwright on the TV show *Bonanza*.

After fourteen years of college and residency, Dr. Bob moved back to Warren to establish his practice in dermatology and picked right up where his father left off, volunteering with the Society first as an educator, then being "sucked in" to do more.

But it was a different Society from the one his father had known. The attendance at the annual meetings of the Trumbull County chapter had dwindled from three hundred down to a handful; one meeting had only twelve attendees. The Society was dying in Trumbull County, despite the best efforts of loyal volunteers who kept searching for new ways to involve the public and raise money. They'd tried gimmicky events, auctions, even a Handsome Hunk contest (which Dr. Bob won) that routinely netted a few thousand dollars.

Now, in 1994, Dr. Bob was at a national meeting of the Society in Florida. Among the workshops the Society was offering on fundraising ideas was a session on three-on-three basketball, and Brodell was eager to get there. Before he went to that one, though, the Society had him scheduled from 9 to 10 a.m. to learn about something called Relay For Life. The description of the session said there'd be a video showing all these people walking around a track for twenty-four hours.

Brodell was pretty sour about the whole idea; it sounded ridiculous to him, even outrageous to waste his time when he could be getting information on three-on-three.

Then he saw the video. Prepared by a television news anchor in Virginia named Terry Zahn, it was stunning.

Zahn had focused his camera on the Hampton Roads, Virginia, Relay that he had helped start, capturing the evocative, emotional phenomenon spawned in Tacoma. Pat Flynn and Gordy Klatt had done a tremendous job on the second annual run/walk in Tacoma in 1986. They called it "The City of Destiny Classic 24-Hour Run Against Cancer." It featured nineteen teams, which collectively raised thirty-three thousand dollars. Every year after that, it just kept getting bigger. Other communities started hearing about the event and were calling Dr. Klatt to ask questions. He began taking time off from his medical practice, traveling to other states to tell his 24-Hour Run Against Cancer story. It wasn't hard to convince the towns and cities to start Relays. "Relays were creating a community. It had developed into a very therapeutic and healing event," says Dr. Klatt.

The Relays were already active in a handful of states before word even made it back to the Society's National Home Office that money—lots more than galas and golf tournaments and charity bike rides raised—was coming in from a

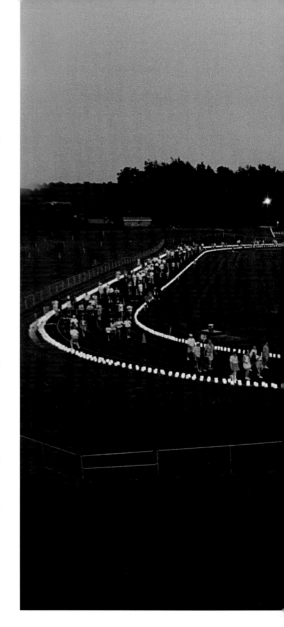

"Relays were creating a community. It had developed into a very therapeutic and healing event."

— Dr. Gordy Klatt

Above: A Relay For Life event
Opposite: A Relay For Life event
in Puerto Rico

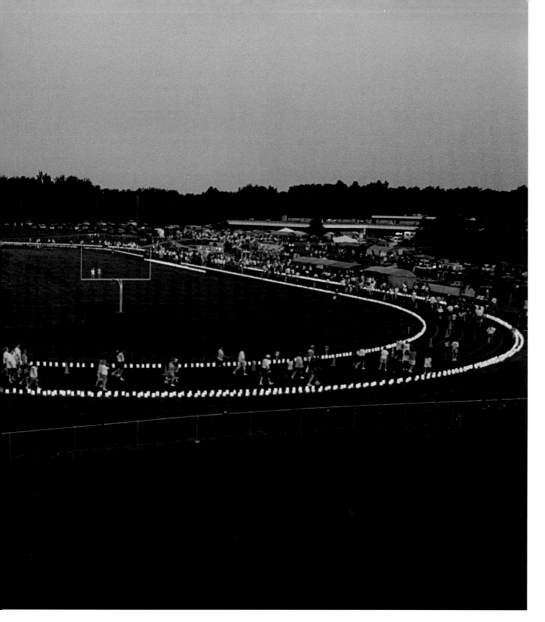

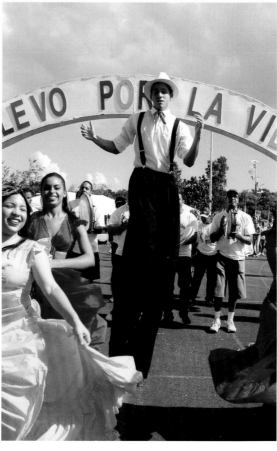

few states holding twenty-four-hour run/walks. It was the grassroots of all grassroots efforts: between 1985 and 1991, before being officially embraced by national, the Relays raised two and a half million dollars.

The Society, trying to get a handle on what was happening, invited Pat Flynn and Gordy Klatt to a national meeting in Nashville, Tennessee, to talk to a special-events breakout group. The Society was understandably dubious. Klatt and Flynn kept using the word "community" when they described the Relays, and Society staff took that to mean that these strange hybrid races could only work in rural areas. Nonetheless, seeing the possibilities, they decided in 1992 to make Relay For Life into the Society's signature event. Klatt and Flynn were asked to be on the design team to work out the plans for everything from the logo to the evening's format—Dr. Klatt to talk about the vision and Pat Flynn the details.

The design team met in a Chicago

hotel conference room at a table packed with marketers. Some of them knew about Relay, some didn't. All of them wanted to talk about target marketing and making things a little slicker.

Flynn and Klatt looked at each other. Target audience? That was anyone who has been touched by cancer. Young? Old? Rich? Poor? Clearly, these folks didn't understand. Relay, they said, was a whole lot more than just people walking around a track. "Relay is not like any event you've ever taken part in," they told the national staff. "There is a feeling of community, a spirit, that appeals to any age, very sick people, very healthy people." They were, in fact, people like Gordy and Pat— Gordy, a tall, lean marathoner, and Pat, a short, size-eighteen community activist. His mother had died of cancer. Her grandmother had died of cancer.

What else was there to say?

"Part of the selling of Relay was just internal," acknowledges Reuel Johnson, who for ten years has run the business side of Relay. "We had to convince people internally that this was the way, that it was a celebration of hope, that it would be a great opportunity to develop leaders on the volunteer side."

"It's Just Magic"

A few people didn't take much convincing,

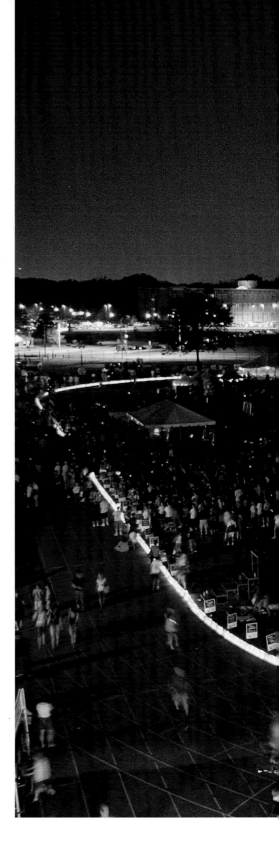

Terry Zahn

such as Terry Zahn, a prominent and popular broadcast journalist in Virginia Beach, Virginia. Zahn's mother was a cancer survivor, and he was very active in the Society. He served as chairman of his local Relay For Life, which at the time was the largest in America. Zahn approached Relay with a ferocious enthusiasm. If you go to the events knowing nobody, he said, you leave knowing everybody on a first-name basis. "I like to call it 'Woodstock without the sex, drugs, and rock 'n' roll,'" he said. "People keep coming back because it's such a neat experience. It's just magic."

In 1993, Zahn produced the first film for the Society to promote Relays. Four years later, he was diagnosed with multiple myeloma, a rare form of bone cancer, and he produced a personal documentary called *My Race Against Cancer* to help raise awareness for the fight against cancer. He produced one more film for the Society on Relay in 1999 and was invited to present the video in person in cities across the country.

Terry Zahn died in January 2000. Each year, the Society presents the Terry Zahn Award for Excellence in Communications to an event that demonstrates a "best practice" in Relay marketing or communication. Upon his death, the Virginia legislature presented a commemorative joint resolution, noting that

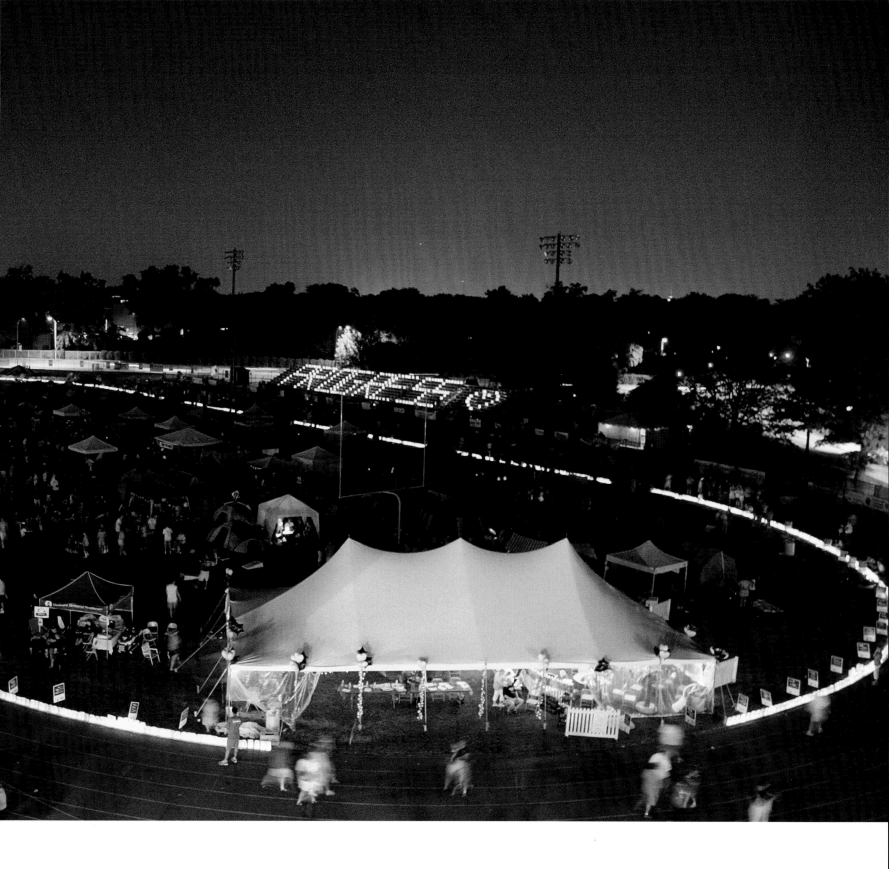

Zahn's "relentless optimistic and positive attitude in the midst of a fight for his life was an inspiration."

Zahn's first Relay For Life film had wowed Dr. Bob in Florida in 1994. Meanwhile, the video had equally inspired volunteer Phylecia Wilson. She had been involved with the American Cancer Society in Gwinnett County, the second-largest county in Georgia, since the 1970s, when a neighbor had asked her to work on one of the community American Cancer Society Crusades. Gwinnett, now a bedroom community of Atlanta, was a heavily rural county at that time, and the Society was having trouble finding women to help with special events. Wilson, along with her friend Bonnie Rose Simmons, agreed to dress up in a dragon costume and go into the elementary schools to show a film about the impact of smoking. After that, she became involved in time-consuming events that raised very little money. One of them, a Jail and Bail—where a community member was "arrested" at a public meeting and taken to a makeshift jail until a friend would come to "bail" them out with a donation—drew a scathing article in the local newspaper. In 1993, a friend, commiserating with Wilson, suggested what they should really be doing was what he called a twenty-four-hour walk.

Phylecia Wilson didn't know what he was talking about, but tracked down some information at the Society's National Home Office in Atlanta. When she saw the video,

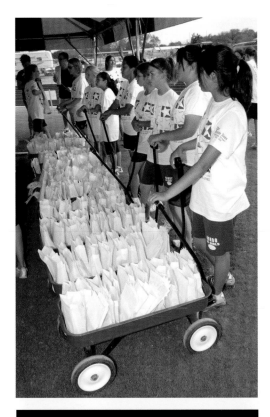

she was "totally sold on it." She asked to cochair a Relay in Gwinnett in 1993. The first year, the goal was forty-three thousand dollars and the event raised one hundred twenty-five thousand; the next year, the goal was two hundred thousand dollars and they raised two hundred fifty thousand. "People still didn't understand Relay," Wilson says, pointing out that she had been urged not to set a goal that year of two hundred thousand because "we were setting ourselves up for failure."

After seeing Zahn's film in 1994, Dr. Bob had rushed back home to tell the people of Trumbull County about Relay, scheduling a meeting of the local board and showing them the video. He and the board planned their first Relay for six weeks later, and went step by step down a list the Society had given him for how to put on a Relay. He went for what he calls the "low-hanging fruit," the people he thought would be sympathetic: his plumber, his neighbors, and his best friend. Trumbull County had fourteen teams and raised twenty-eight thousand dollars that first Relay; in 2005, there were five Relays in Trumbull County, and they raised $1.3 million. Dr. Bob's team alone raised fifty thousand dollars.

"Every person whose arm I ever twisted is glad to come back," he says. His entire family—including his wife, an ophthalmologist, and his five children—has been involved with Relay. His daughter, Lindsey, even started the largest college Relay when she attended Washington University in St. Louis, Missouri, raising two hundred sixty thousand dollars for the Society.

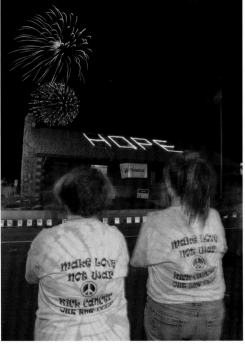

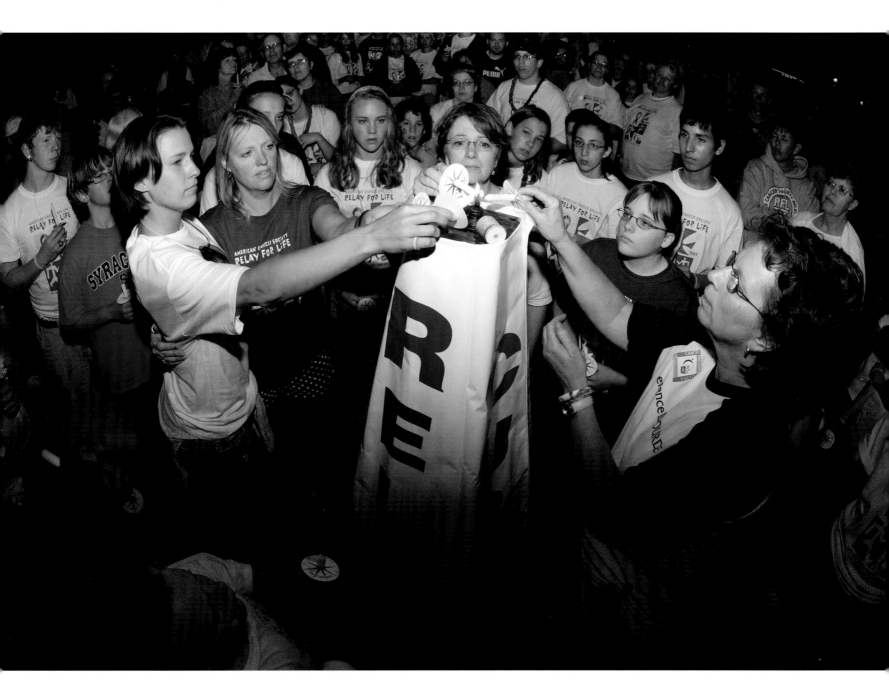

Opposite top: Volunteers at a Relay event

Opposite bottom: Fireworks at a Relay event

Above: Lighting candles at a Relay event

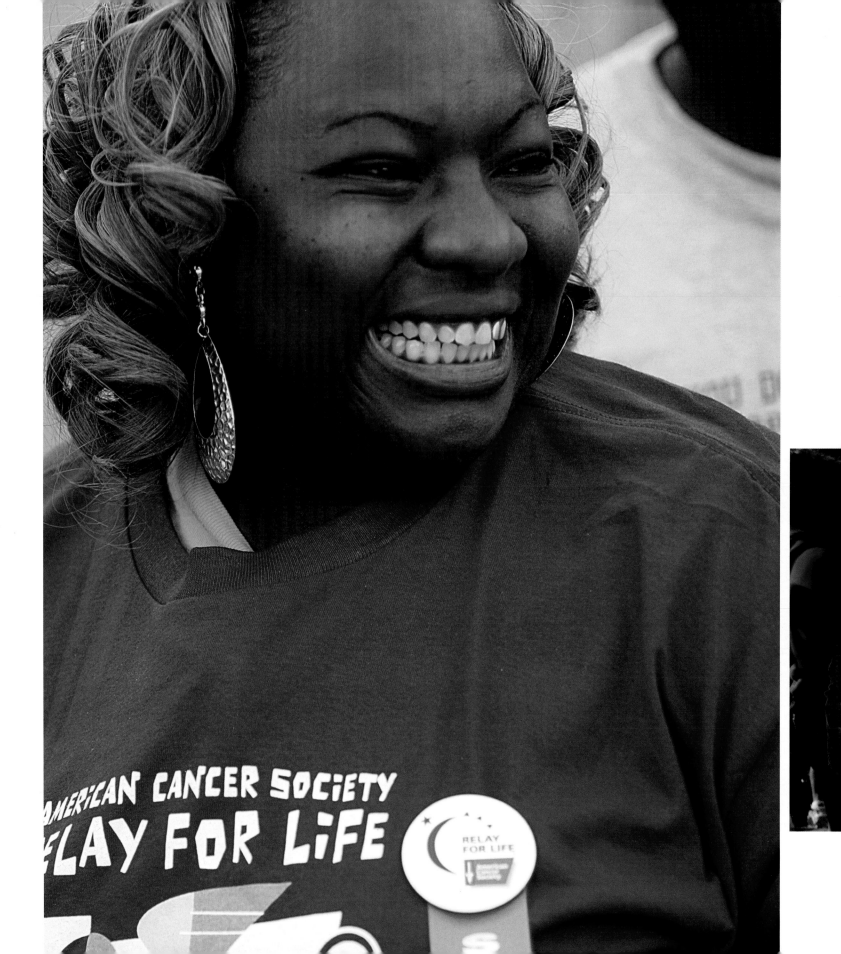

"As long as there is a way, I will walk, talk, and donate for a day and a world free from cancer."
— Laura Wilson, Relayer

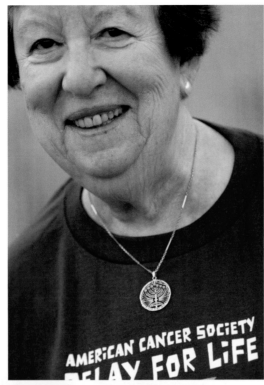

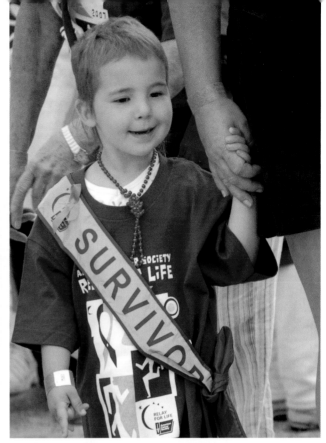

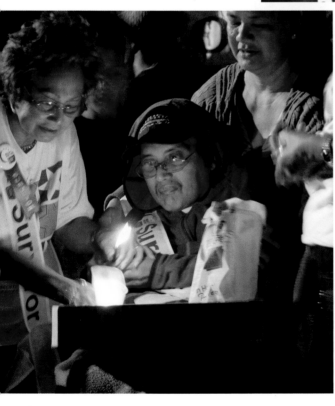

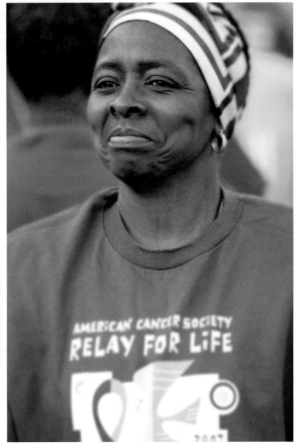

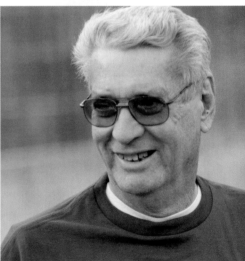

Different—but the Same

Relay For Life has gone through many changes since 1985. That first one had no luminaria, no Survivors Lap, no teams, and no tents, and it was twenty-four hours long. Today's Relays are overnight events, lasting from twelve to twenty-four hours. Teams of people camp out at a local high school, park, or fairground and take turns walking or running around a track or path. Participants also have the opportunity to learn about cancer prevention and the Society's programs and services for survivors and caregivers. In 2007, the Relays also became the starting point for the Society's third Cancer Prevention Study (CPS-3), in which five hundred thousand Relay participants are being asked to participate in a long-range study to gather new information on cancer development and prevention.

Relay For Life participants are also the basis for a powerful grassroots organization. Relays are a source of attendees of the Celebration on the Hill™, a remarkable event held in 2002 and again in 2006 in Washington, D.C., to demonstrate the voting power and reach of cancer survivors (see Chapter 9, "Powerful Friends").

Some things, though, have not changed.

Gordy Klatt still walks each year. To recognize his work, volunteers in Tacoma honored him by establishing the Relay For Life Gordon Klatt Research Endowment Fund to support research. Gordy and his wife, Lou, made the first commitment to the

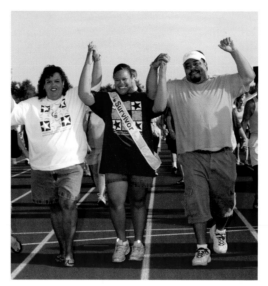

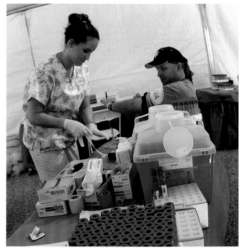

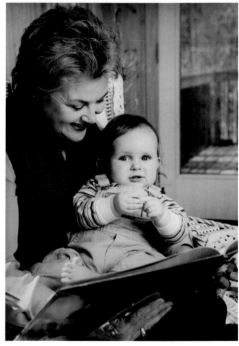

endowment. Pat Flynn captains a family team and is usually in the top five fundraisers. Dr. Bob still competes every year with his plumber and friend, Robert Antenucci, to see who can raise the most at that year's Relay; Antenucci himself has become a most willing captive of the Society, holding every position in the Trumbull County chapter. He was in charge of the luminaria ceremony at the 2006 Celebration on the Hill. Phylecia Wilson takes her own Survivors Lap now. She was diagnosed in 2001 with chronic myeloid leukemia and was placed a few months later into a clinical trial for a new drug called Gleevec, invented by researcher Dr. Brian Druker, who received his first grant money from the Society. While Wilson walks, she thinks about her two uncles, who died of lung cancer; her aunt, who died of colon cancer; and Bonnie Rose Simmons, her old dragon partner and best friend, who died of uterine cancer on the morning of her fortieth birth-

Top left: Relay participants. Top: A volunteer has blood drawn as part of Cancer Prevention Study-3. Above: Phylecia Wilson helped launch Relay in Gwinnett County, Georgia, hoping to raise forty-three thousand dollars the first year in 1993. They raised three times that amount. Opposite: Participants for a Relay get animated for the camera. It's not uncommon for lifelong friends to be made at the events.

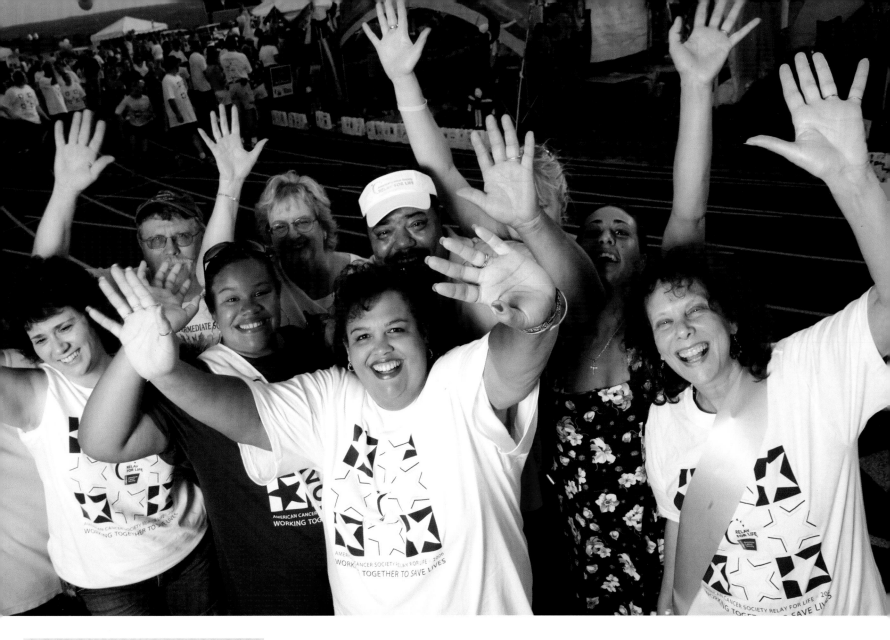

day—more than two decades ago. Wilson still celebrates that birthday every year for Bonnie.

Each of them will tell you the same thing: You can't explain Relay. You must experience it. As Relay founder Dr. Klatt puts it, "Human beings all react the same when they're touched by this disease."

Laura Wilson of Lilburn, Georgia, probably describes it best. In her lifetime, she has lost two sons to cancer, one when he was only five, one when he was twenty-three. For years, she has participated in Relay For Life; after she walked as a team member in the 2006 Gwinnett County Relay For Life she wrote, "As long as there is a way, I will walk, talk, and donate for a day and a world free from cancer."

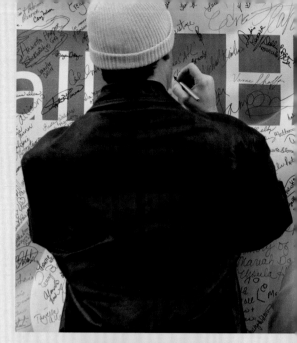

MAKING STRIDES AGAINST BREAST CANCER

In 1984, non-Hodgkin lymphoma survivor Margery "Margie" Gould Rath wanted to find a way to give back to her community and show her appreciation for the support she had received during her own battle with cancer. The idea of a fundraising walk appealed to Margie—participants could walk at their own pace rather than compete against each other. The event would celebrate fellow cancer survivors and also raise money for the American Cancer Society. With the help of other survivors and volunteers, she pioneered the first Making Strides Against Cancer event, held in Boston, Massachusetts. More than two hundred people participated in the fundraiser, which became an annual event for the city.

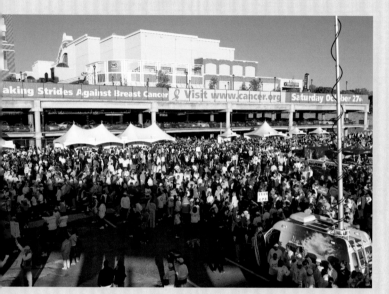

In 1993, the event officially became known as the American Cancer Society Making Strides Against Breast Cancer®, attracting four thousand walkers. Today, Making Strides Against Breast Cancer is the American Cancer Society's premier event to raise awareness and funds to fight breast cancer. As of 2008, nearly five million walkers had raised more than three hundred and forty million dollars through Making Strides events across the country. In 2008 alone, nearly six hundred thousand walkers collected more than sixty million dollars.

The majority of Making Strides events take place in October, National Breast Cancer Awareness Month. The events rally people of all ages. The average distance of the walk is five miles, and participants can take as long as they need to finish or walk as far as they are able.

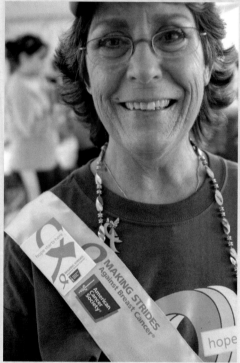

The money raised through Making Strides funds cutting-edge research and helps the American Cancer Society provide valuable services to patients and their families. Support services include the state-of-the-art Web site www.cancer.org; the National Cancer Information Center's twenty-four-hour hotline; and programs for patients and survivors, such as Reach to Recovery®, a service that matches newly diagnosed breast cancer patients with breast cancer survivors who can help guide them through their breast cancer journey by providing information and emotional support.

"When you see thousands of people walking for this cause, you can't help but feel the passion and the hope—the hope that one day, we will walk together to celebrate the fact that breast cancer no longer threatens those we love," says Alix Shaer, ACS National Making Strides director. "Until that day, we will continue to have Making Strides Against Breast Cancer to support all people with breast cancer—before, during, and after diagnosis. That's why there is Making Strides."

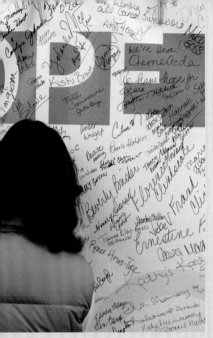

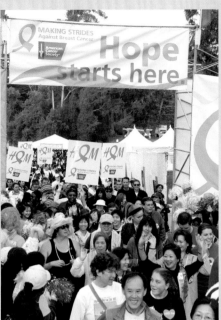

"When we got to the Making Strides event, there were tents, music, and thousands of people. It was amazing. I was so proud to be a survivor. I never felt so happy to be alive."

—Judy Gloden,
breast cancer survivor
and Making Strides team leader

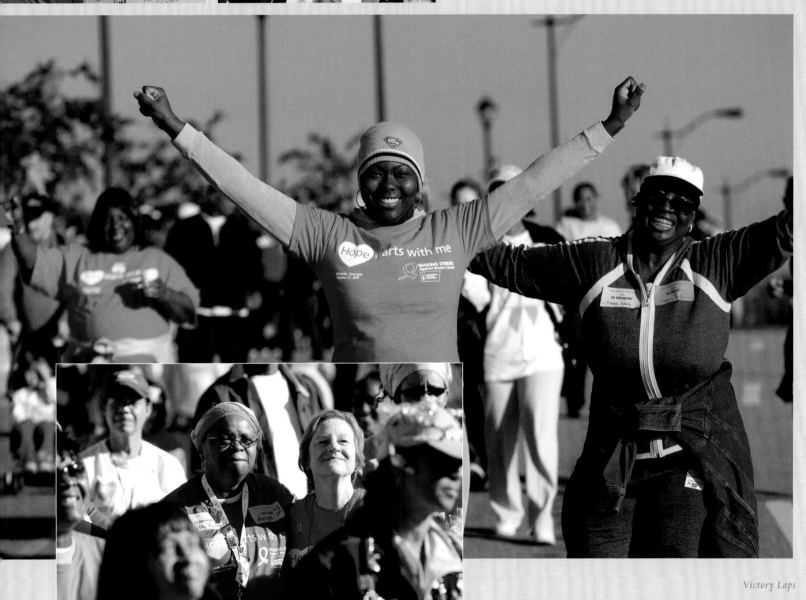

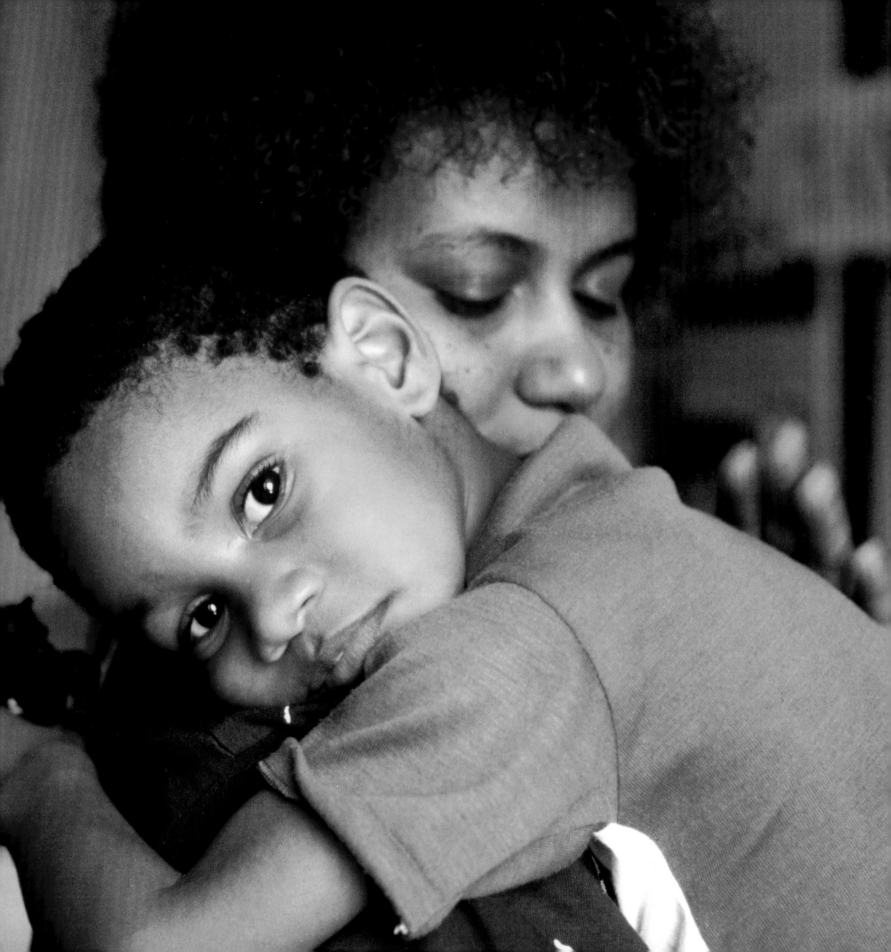

The Warm Hand of Service

The early days of the American Cancer Society had been marked by its commitment to education and service. The Society still draws on those early roots, providing information and programs that help millions of patients and their families and friends learn about, cope with, and make informed decisions about prevention, diagnosis, treatment, and recovery. The programs and information the Society provides to cancer patients and their families have been its most defining elements over the years—what Lane Adams, the top Society leader for twenty-six years, labeled almost four decades ago as the Society's "warm hand of service."

If you've decided to quit smoking, if you need a ride to your cancer treatments, if you're looking for advice on the foods you can keep down during chemotherapy, if you want to meet with other survivors for hope and support, if you need information on the latest research or clinical trials on a loved one's type of cancer, or just need someone to talk to at 2 a.m., the American Cancer Society is there to help.

The Society was the first to launch a twenty-four-hour, seven-day-a-week National Cancer Information Center, which regularly fields more than one million calls a year and more than four thousand e-mails a month from people looking for information about cancer. The Society was the first to launch a phone-in smokers' cessation program (see sidebar, right), the first to connect patients to a survivor-to-survivor support program for breast cancer patients, the first to recognize that everyone needs to look good and feel better while undergoing cancer treatments, and the first to provide temporary housing to cancer patients and their families who must leave home to receive proper treatment.

The names of many of these programs are now an integral part of the fabric of the Society—Hope Lodge®, Reach to Recovery®, I Can Cope®, Road to Recovery®, Quitline®, Great American Smokeout®, Man to Man®, "tlc" Tender Loving Care®, Look Good . . . Feel Better®, the National Cancer Information Center—and remain a primary part of the Society's work to meet its mission. After its support of research, they are the programs for which the Society is best known, the lifeblood that not only feeds it as a health care organization but also provides the warm hand of service for those in need. Many of these programs were also a direct outgrowth of community support for the Society, originating from the ground up: the Illinois Division was the first to have a cancer information hotline (the Cancer Response System, begun in 1984), The Great American Smokeout came from a Minnesota newspaper publisher who urged "D-Day" (for "don't smoke") on his hometown of Monticello in 1974, and Reach to Recovery started as one woman's attempt to share with other women what she'd learned after her mastectomy.

These quality-of-life programs have served hundreds of thousands of people who have either made use of the services themselves or who have volunteered for them, as a vital and personal way of contributing to the fight against cancer.

They are people like Margot Freudenberg, a Holocaust survivor who lives in Charleston, South Carolina. In the late 1960s, she traveled to New Zealand as part of a program started by President Dwight D. Eisenhower called People to People. There, she saw a facility for cancer patients and caregivers called Hope Lodge. She returned to the United States and asked Charleston business leaders to help open a Hope Lodge there in 1970. In 2009, there were twenty-eight American Cancer Society Hope Lodge facilities around the country providing free, temporary housing for cancer patients who are undergoing treatment away from home.

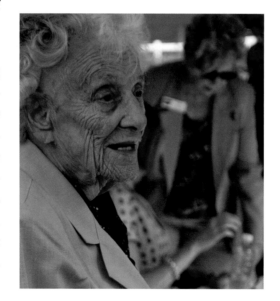

Left: Margot Freudenberg, founder of the Hope Lodge movement in the United States. At 102, Margot is the longest-serving volunteer in the American Cancer Society. She arrived in Charleston, South Carolina, in 1940 as a survivor from Nazi Germany, and spent her life working tirelessly for a long list of charitable causes. "I have got so much satisfaction and happiness by trying to help people in distress," she told the Charleston News and Courier in 1959. "This is my repaying of my debt [to America]." Opposite top left: A warm welcome at Florida's Winn-Dixie Hope Lodge. Opposite top right: Hope Lodge in Worcester, Massachusetts. Opposite bottom: Guests in the greenhouse at a New York Hope Lodge

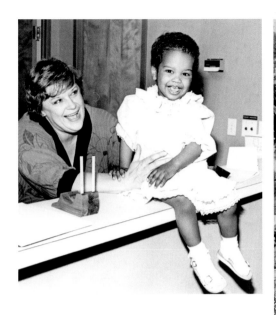

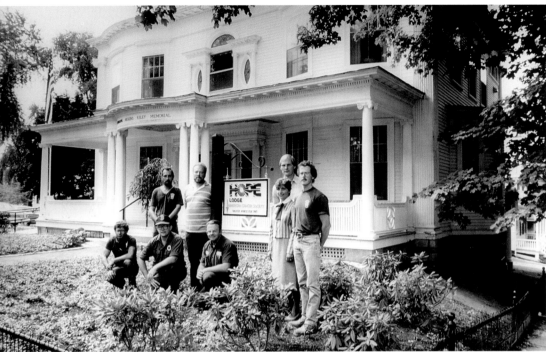

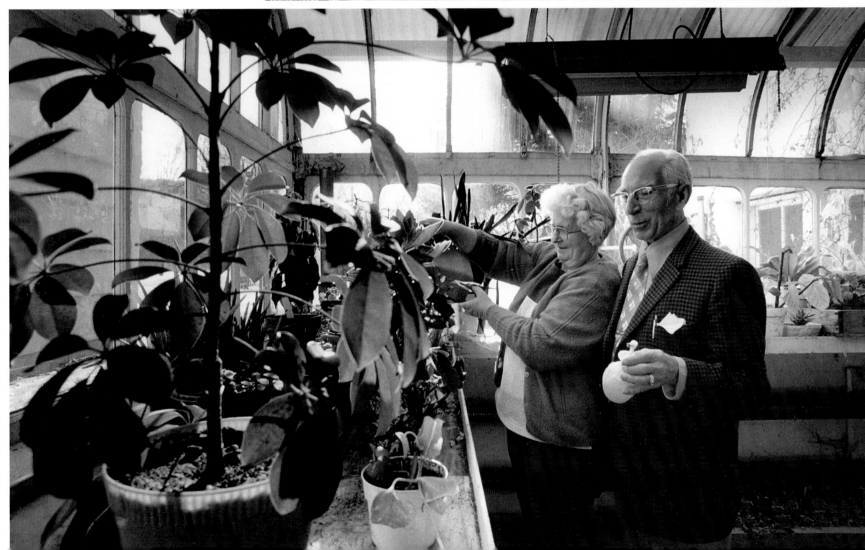

They are people like Stephen Mallane, who owns a hair salon in Johnston, Rhode Island, and first knew the Society through its Look Good . . . Feel Better program, a collaboration between the Cosmetic, Toiletry, and Fragrance Association, the National Cosmetology Association, and the American Cancer Society. Look Good . . . Feel Better is a free, nationwide public service program helping patients undergoing chemotherapy and radiation treatments learn how to cope with the appearance-related side effects of their treatment. After Mallane was able to help people through Look Good . . . Feel Better, he realized he, too, was feeling better—and became an organizer of his community's Relay For Life.

They are people like Deborah Cornwall, a Boston businesswoman who had served on the Society's New England Division board for years when she was diagnosed with breast cancer during a routine mammogram, one of the prevention tests the Society had helped develop and promote more than twenty years earlier. Thunderstruck by the diagnosis—but also lucky enough to have been diagnosed early—she decided to step up her involvement with the Society, serving as an ambassador at Celebration on the Hill and as the Massachusetts spokesperson who asked U.S. Senator Edward "Ted" Kennedy to sign the Congressional Cancer Promise (see Chapter 9, "Powerful Friends"). Her adult daughter, a civil rights attorney, called just before Celebration to tell her mother how much she admired her for her work with the

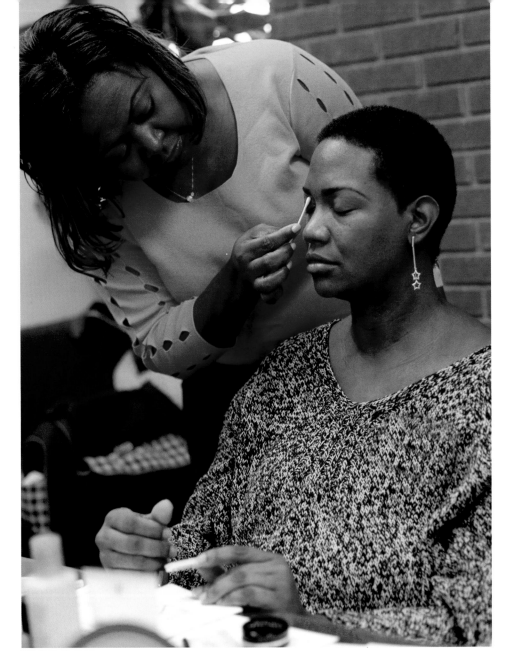

Society. "I never knew you'd get so involved and make such a difference."

They are people, too, like Brandi Jagemann of Montpelier, Vermont. She was twenty-four, married less than a year, and eighteen weeks pregnant with her first child when she was diagnosed with lymphocytic leukemia in February 2003. She had no known

Above: The Society's free Look Good . . . Feel Better program helps women cope with appearance-related issues from cancer treatment. Opposite: At Duke University Medical Center, a patient applies makeup as cosmetologist Cindy Ruth demonstrates technique.

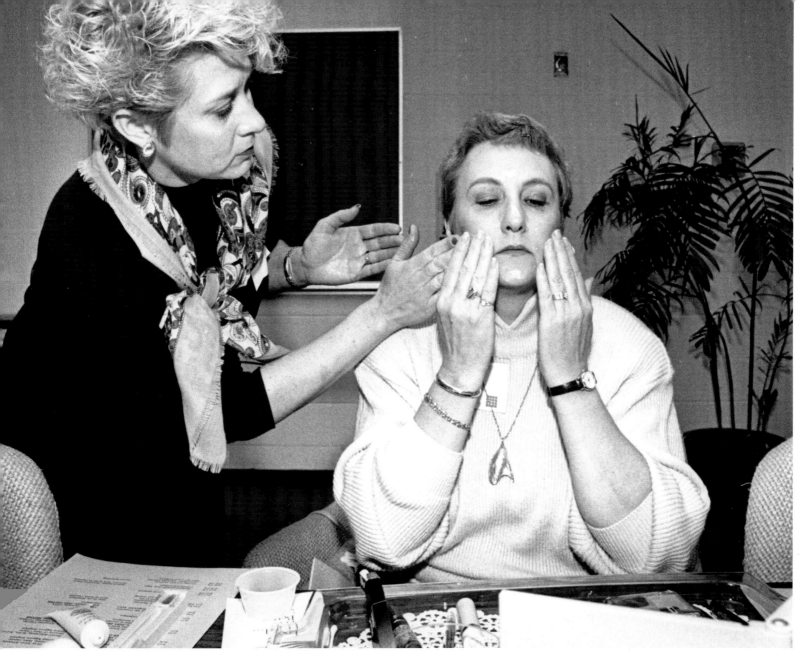

risk factors and no symptoms except tiredness. She and her husband, a political science professor at Norwich University, had already picked out the name for their daughter. During her pregnancy, Jagemann spent twenty-two days in the hospital, underwent twenty bone marrow treatments, and lost all her hair—twice. Immediately after the birth of her daughter, Jaeden, she began eighteen months of maintenance chemotherapy.

Jagemann credits the American Cancer Society with her life. Were it not for the research it supported to find a treatment for leukemia, she might not be alive; and certainly, five years earlier, she would have had to decide whether to save her own life or her unborn

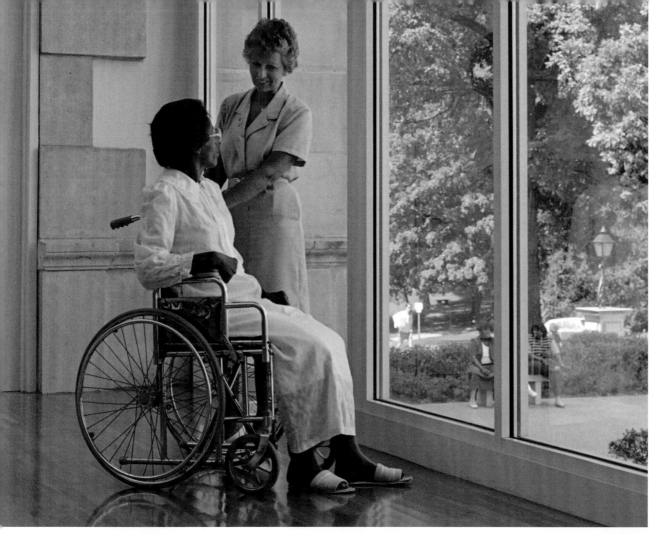

Left: A cancer patient receives personal attention from a nurse. Bottom left: Divisions and Units of the Society provided service to cancer patients by supplying special equipment and dressings. Bottom right: A volunteer demonstrates how to unfold a bed tray.

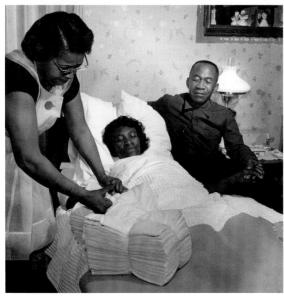

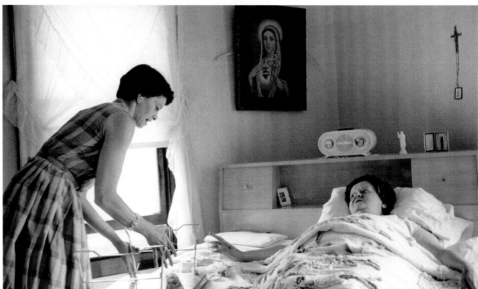

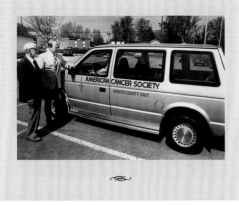

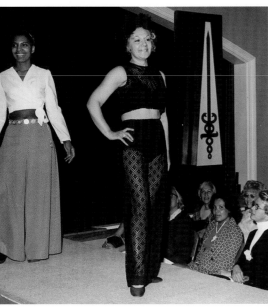

Above: A fashion show staged by the Philadelphia Division in 1973 by and for breast cancer survivors. All the models were women who had had mastectomies.

child's. While Jagemann was hospitalized, her best friend, Megan, called the Society's hotline regularly and passed information on to Jagemann and her husband, Jason. Not a "support-group-type person," Jagemann has long since overcome her hesitancy to reach out to the Society for help. She helped begin a Road to Recovery program in her community as soon as she was healthy. She was an ambassador at the second Celebration on the Hill event in Washington, D.C. In large part, she tells her story to remind people, "Those of us who owe our lives to research have names and faces." She had her second child, a son named Jackson, in 2006.

After all she has learned, she has returned to college to become a nurse.

Saying Thanks

It has long been recognized that information and advice about prevention, health care, and treatment is often passed from friend to friend, neighbor to neighbor—at the water cooler, across the pew, or over the fence.

Patricia Swanson couldn't talk over her fence. She lives in the northwest corner of Minnesota twenty miles from Canada, on a grain and soybean farm between two tiny towns named Hallock and Kennedy, and her neighbors are too far away for fence-chatting. Yet she is the type of woman the Society recognizes as a natural leader in the fight against cancer, the type to help start and run cancer survivor programs in her community.

Swanson is a hospice nurse who, as she says, "looked this ugly disease in the face for years" before she became directly involved with the Society. She became president of her local Unit in 1976 in a moment of desperation, when it didn't have a president and one of the local Society supporters asked her to take the job for one year. She arrived at her first meeting both as a new volunteer and as president—and stayed for two decades.

During that time, she helped start a run/walk dedicated to a young woman who had died of cancer in 1981, and eventually turned that into a Relay For Life event. She helped coproduce and codirect three concerts to benefit the Society. She began a Fall Style Show and a "Superball" youth basketball tournament that has been an annual event since 1978.

Her "little" Kittson County Unit, in an area with a population of just under five thousand, received a national Society award in 1990 for being the highest-per-capita unit in contributions in the country. Since 1978, those donations have ranged from seven dollars to nine dollars per capita each year. Swanson describes the appreciation of the "wonderful, generous people" of Kittson County for the work the Society does in their community. "They are quick to express their appreciation of our educational efforts that have saved the lives of their family members, the materials we provide our medical professionals, and the immense progress we have made in research over the years."

They are grateful that the Society helps make life better.

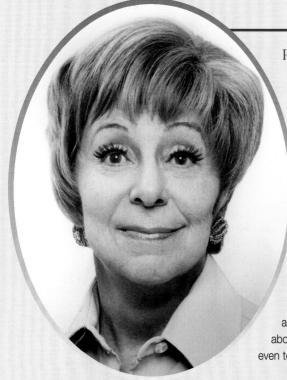

Terese Lasser

REACH TO RECOVERY

They threw Terese Lasser out of the hospital when they found her giving advice to other women, told her no layperson should be seeing patients, escorted her to the door, and told her not to come back.

Lasser—the wife of a famous tax expert, a woman who loved dancing, swimming, golf, and parties—was forty-eight when her doctor discovered a small lump in her right breast in 1952. He scheduled her for a routine biopsy, which entailed a hospital stay. Doctors would get a reading on the biopsy at the time it was done: if it was cancerous, they would immediately remove the affected breast, the lymph nodes in the chest and under the arm, and muscle tissue. Lasser was so unconcerned about the potential for that happening that she hadn't even told her husband.

When she woke from the anesthesia, she found herself in agony, bandaged from the midriff to the neck, feeling suddenly like half a woman. No one could tell her what the next step was— how to make her clothes hang right, what sort of exercises she could do to counteract the surgery, and what, and how, to tell her husband about what had just happened to her.

As Lasser stumblingly began to heal herself and deal with her new body, she found other women in the same situation. She began to carry a little handmade kit she'd made, with ropes and balls and even a lightweight breast form a woman could pin inside her nightgown so they could receive visitors looking the way they always had. At first, she ruffled a lot of feathers, including some at the American Cancer Society. Dr. A. Hamblin Letton, a well-known surgeon from Georgia who became president of the Society in 1972, remembers a woman from Connecticut on the Society's education committee, pointing out that a mastectomy is a defeminizing procedure that no man could understand. Only a woman who had gone through the procedure, she told him, could help another woman. Letton managed to bring peace between Lasser and the Society; in 1969, Reach to Recovery became a sanctioned Society program.

The program connects trained volunteers—themselves breast cancer survivors—with patients and family members, giving them an opportunity to express feelings, talk about fears and concerns, and ask questions of someone who is knowledgeable and levelheaded. Most important, Reach to Recovery volunteers offer understanding, support, and hope because they themselves have survived breast cancer and gone on to live normal, productive lives.

It was the first survivor-to-survivor program ever introduced for breast cancer patients, and it remains a model today for programs serving patients with many forms of cancer.

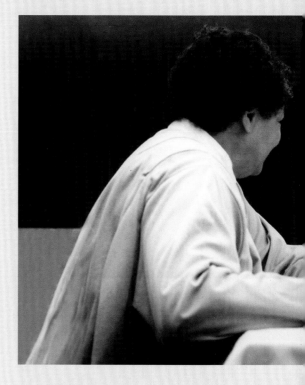

Above: A Reach to Recovery volunteer and a patient. Above right: Mrs. Terese Lasser, in an impromptu meeting with leaders in cancer control at the Manila, Philippines, airport shortly after Lasser arrived for a tour through the Far East. Opposite bottom: Terese Lasser in Nagoya, Japan, where she conducted a workshop with physicians and lay leaders in cancer control, explaining the important features of Reach to Recovery

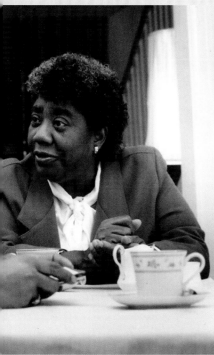

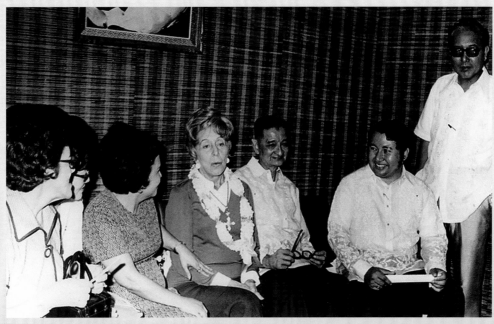

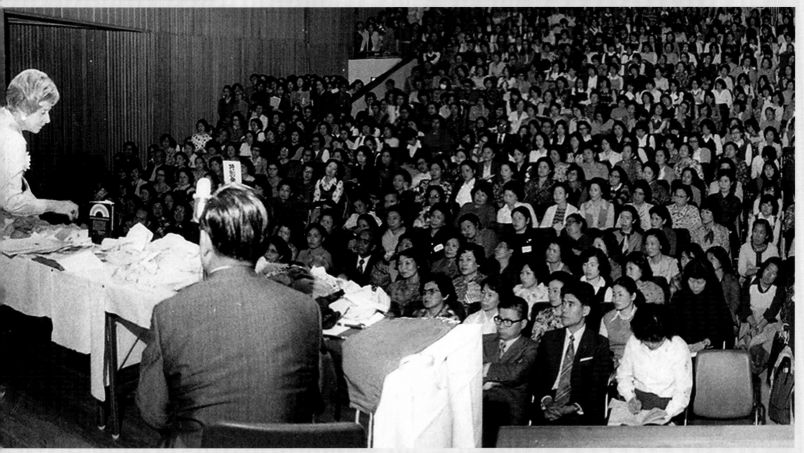

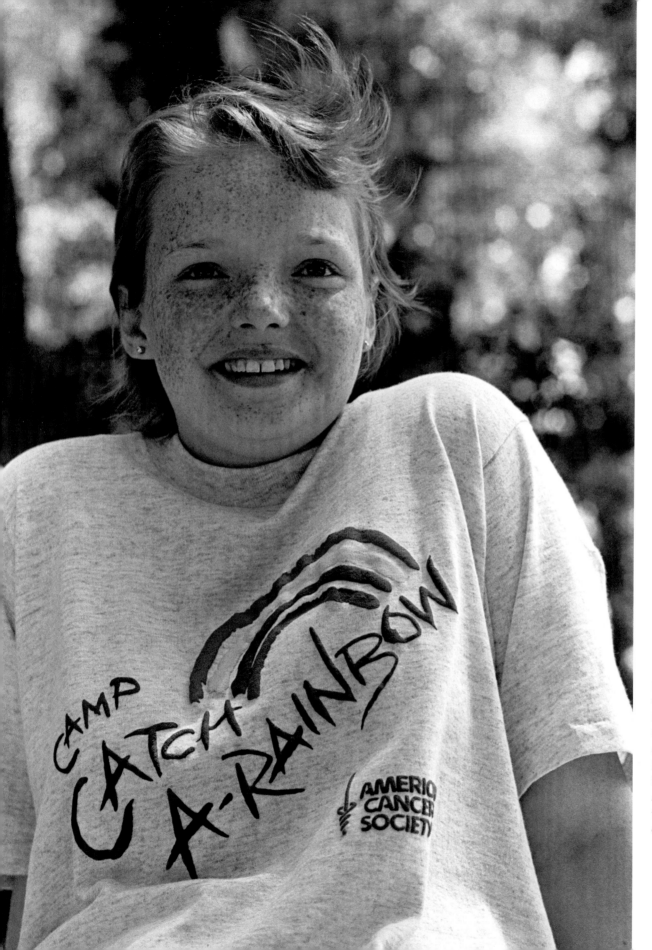

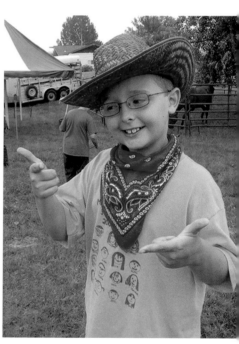

"Camp Hope means getting together with a lot of other people who don't think you're weird. They're different themselves."

— Hailey Rago,
diagnosed at age nine with
medulloblastoma,
a type of brain tumor

Left: Camper Charlene Dawson at Camp Catch-A-Rainbow, a program of the then Michigan Division of the Society. Camp Catch-A-Rainbow was one of many camps that have been sponsored by the Society over the years for children who have or have recovered from cancer.

Above: Camper Mike Underdown, ready for a day of horseback riding at a Society camp facility

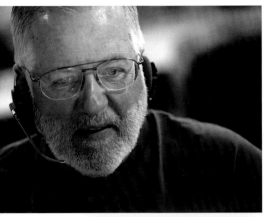

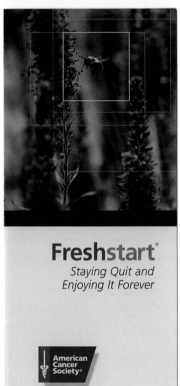

Freshstart
*Staying Quit and
Enjoying It Forever*

Top: A Cancer Information Specialist at the American Cancer Society's National Cancer Information Center in Austin, Texas.
Above: A Society publication about quitting tobacco

One Mission, One Voice: The Information Age

From its founding, the Society had been grounded in a profound commitment to providing accurate, clear information to the public. That commitment had been reaffirmed in the early 1990s with the board's adoption of the five strategic directions, and, in particular, the first of those directions: the Society's continued commitment to leadership in the development and delivery of cancer information.

The state of information delivery nationwide at the Society in the early 1990s was fractured at best and did not reflect the innovations in technology that were exploding around the world. The organization had no uniform quality standards by which it developed and updated its vast library of cancer content. The organization did have a toll-free number, but it was completely decentralized —managed locally by each Division as they could afford to staff and fund it. There were no nationwide standards or consistency regarding how staff fulfilled requests for information or referred patients and caregivers to needed resources.

The Society needed one voice. National leaders recognized the need to pull together the many possible ways of sharing information with the public and the way it managed its stores of

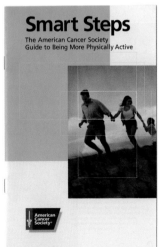

This Society publication touted the benefits of leading an active lifestyle.

information and to develop nationwide strategies to reach patients and families, where, when, and how they needed it most.

Then Chief Operating Officer Don Thomas asked Harry Johns, an executive from the Florida Division, to come to the National Home Office and create a new business unit called Health Content Products. Having spent six years in the Arizona Division and six in Florida, Johns was responsible for creating a call center in Florida that would be the prototype for the Society's new National Cancer Information Center (NCIC). Dr. David Rosenthal (who would later serve as president of the Society in 1998) chaired a committee that oversaw the development of the plan and shepherded it through. Under Johns's and Rosenthal's leadership, the new business unit launched the NCIC, developed a new Web presence at www.cancer.org, and created a professional and consumer publishing program. Driving their efforts was the acknowledgment that cancer information needed to be continually researched and made available to the patient and caregiver, in language that was accessible and easy to understand.

Call Anytime, Day or Night

In January 1997, the American Cancer Society opened the

National Cancer Information Center in Austin, Texas, as a resource for patients for high-quality information, services, and referrals to resources in their community. Since its opening, the NCIC has empowered millions of patients and their families and has become the nation's most trusted resource for cancer information, programs, and services. Terry Music, who came to the National Home Office from the Florida Division to enact the NCIC plan, and is now chief mission delivery officer, recalls those early days:

During the earliest days of the NCIC opening, I have two distinct memories. We had worked with the producers of the television show *Murphy Brown* and had provided them with specific information that used the NCIC as a call to action. During the segment, Murphy was diagnosed with cancer and mentioned the American Cancer Society. The commercial break then aired a Society public service announcement with our toll-free number. As soon as the show aired and the number was shown, the phone lines literally lit up. We stood and watched in amazement as the power of media drove callers to us.

During that same event, we were not yet operating twenty-four/seven, but we had extended the hours to midnight Central Time. However, the call volume really dropped off around 10:30, so we sent most of the Cancer Information Specialists home and the management team began to answer phones. The first caller I spoke with had just been diagnosed with her third cancer and she was very depressed. She wanted to talk and just needed to find a sympathetic ear. As she talked, it also became apparent that she was emotionally distressed and was contemplating suicide. Knowing that I could not provide her with what she needed and also driven by the fact that our system was going to "close" at midnight—literally, the switch was going to cut the phone lines over to the automated answering system—I had to find resources to help her. I knew where she was calling from because the system had captured her area code, and I was frantically writing notes to the staff to find resources for me. . . . They called the area code of her home town and found a 911 service that we could transfer her to. . . . We accomplished the successful handoff with only minutes to spare before the midnight cutoff! I was emotionally exhausted when the call ended, but I immediately recognized what a powerful service we were going to provide to the American public.

On the Web and on the Shelves

The state of the Society's Web presence was

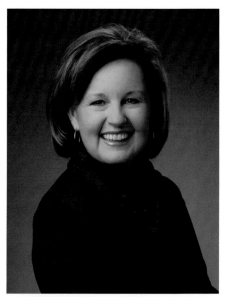

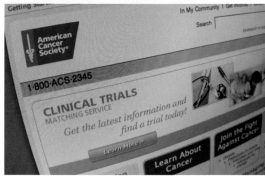

Top: Terry Music came to the National Home Office from the Florida Division to implement the National Cancer Information Center in Austin. She now serves as the Society's chief mission delivery officer. Above: The Society's Web site, www.cancer.org, launched in 1996, was cited by a national business magazine for its extensive information about cancer and clinical trials. It gets tens of thousands of visits per day.

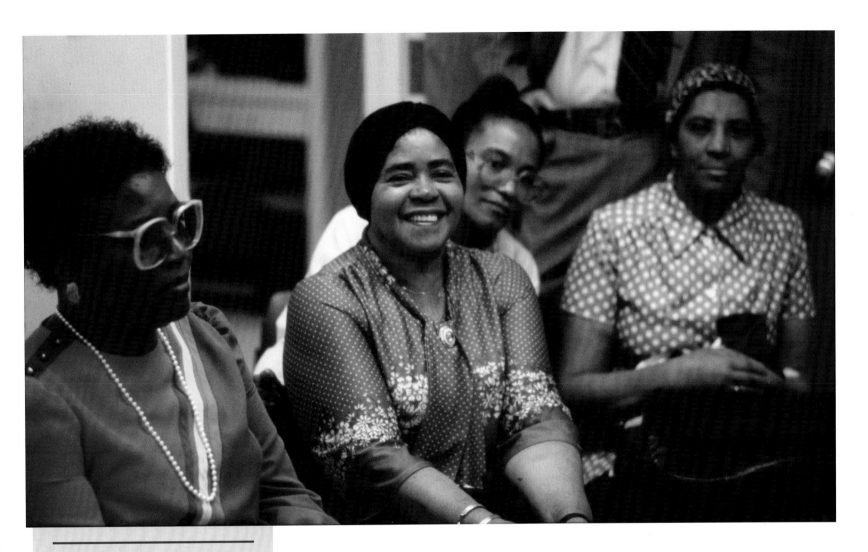

I CAN COPE

The Society has long recognized that living with cancer can be one of the greatest challenges a person can face in the course of a lifetime. I Can Cope® is an educational program for people facing cancer—either in their own life or as a friend or family caregiver. The classes help dispel cancer myths by presenting straightforward facts about diagnosis and treatment, side effects, nutrition, pain management, financial concerns, and the many other areas in which cancer affects one's life.

minimal in 1995. In 1996, the Society launched a new Web site, which was recognized by *Forbes* magazine for its extensive packaging of cancer information, decision tools, and clinical trials information. And the public took notice. The number of visitors to www.cancer.org jumped from about a thousand visits per day to more than sixty-five thousand visits per day in 2009.

The Society continued to establish its leadership in the delivery of cancer informa-tion by broadening its reach into more traditional channels. In 1997, the Society created a publishing program to take the cancer content being developed for the NCIC and Web site and create books for patients and families. A consumer imprint was born, and the first major consumer book, *Informed Decisions*, was published. Since that time, dozens of consumer titles have been published, winning awards such as Best Consumer Health Book by *Library Journal*.

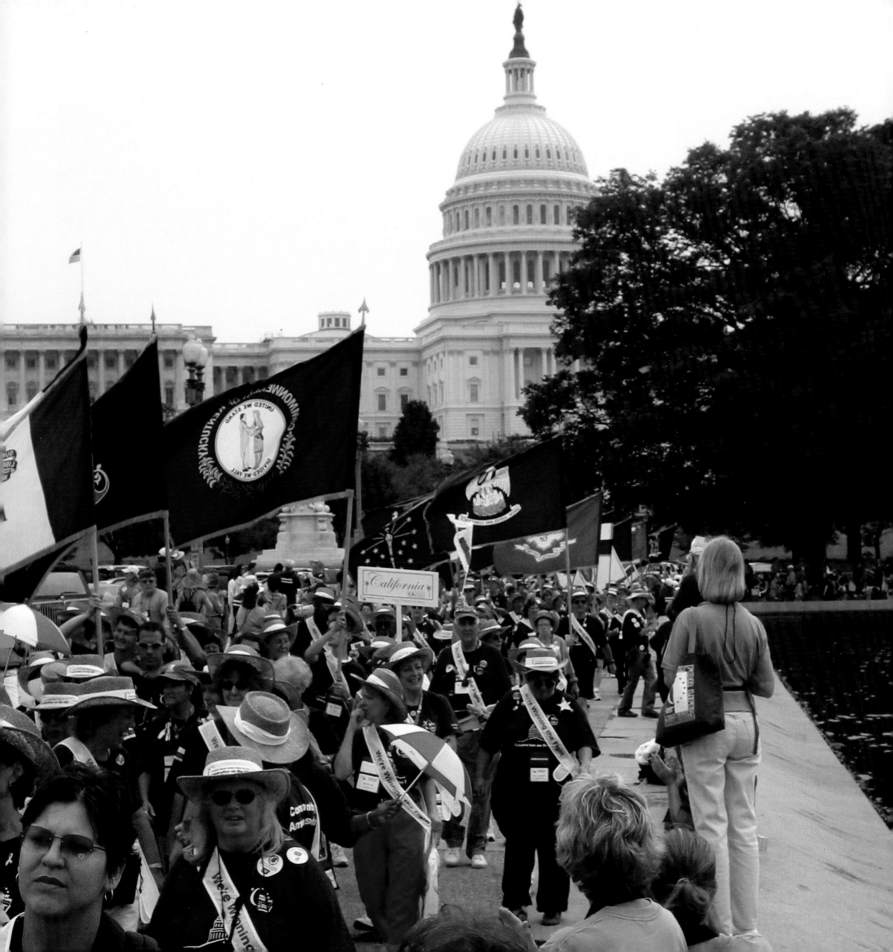

Powerful Friends

CHAPTER NINE

It looked like an army going into battle.

For thirty minutes, wave after wave of men and women, youth and children, flowed around the U.S. Capitol Reflecting Pool, purple t-shirts like punctuation marks against the beige limestone of the walkway and steps surrounding the pool. Sandi and Mary from Nebraska, former strangers, now good friends united by a common disease, were there. Cindy from Missouri, whose body has taken so much punishment, was there. Fourteen-year-old Alex from Massachusetts—with his titanium backbone replacing the one eaten by cancer—and his mom were there. Susan from Rhode Island was there, the disease that would have killed her detected by a persistent doctor. Brandi from Vermont was there, her babies—including the three-year-old she had carried for only eighteen weeks before finding she had leukemia—back home.

Like rock stars, they circled the pool while thousands more stood on the sidelines, cheering and reaching out to slap hands, crying as the crowd in the white sashes imprinted with a single word, "Survivor," moved past them—the tiny children in strollers, the woman with one leg, the teenagers looking mildly embarrassed, the Florida women gently thumbing their noses at the disease with funny hats sporting feathery pink flamingos, the wheelchairs for those who could not walk, the bald ones obviously in chemotherapy. On

Opposite: Celebration on the Hill event in 2002

and on they came, the memories almost too much, the pain too real. The determination was strong, the slogan on the back of all those t-shirts—"We care about cancer and we will be heard"—a blessing for those who listened and a warning for those who didn't.

To their right, as they traveled the east side of the pool, each cancer survivor turned and looked at the imposing white dome where five hundred thirty-five senators and representatives decide a future that might mean life and death to them or to another generation of people like them. What were they thinking, the men and women of Congress for whom this army had been assembled? Did they remember their mothers ("She died in my arms."—Representative William Delahunt; "She was in the prime of her life."—then Senator Barack Obama) or their fathers, sons, daughters, husbands, wives, sisters, brothers, uncles, aunts, best friends, heroes? Did they think of this—as participants in this Celebration on the Hill did—as a war that all America wants to fight? Did they vote with their hearts, signing a promise to fight the good fight for all those who have or will be touched by cancer?

Did they agree to try to make life better?

On this September day in 2006, Celebration on the Hill™ assembled a crowd of almost ten thousand ambassadors and supporters from every congressional district in the country, pitched fifty state tents for them on the long grassy mall leading through the heart of Washington, D.C., from the Capitol to the Washington Monument, put up a modern

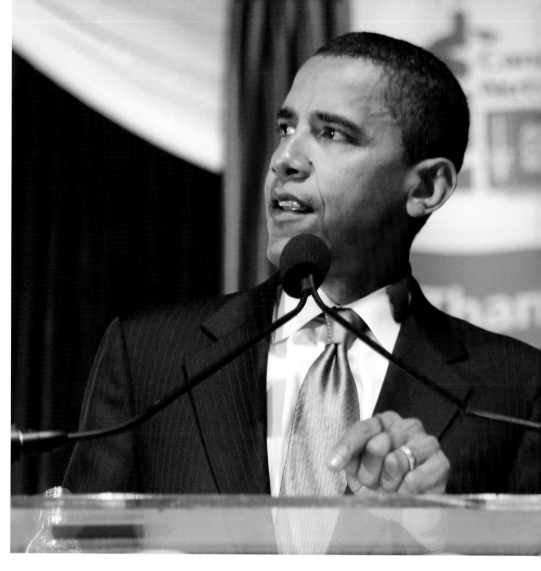

sculpture of five thousand banners fifteen feet high, four city blocks long, and signed by three million people, and made appointments for Celebration on the Hill ambassadors to meet with every U.S. senator and representative. The ambassadors carried with them a pledge sheet asking the national leaders to provide more funding for breast and cervical cancer programs, to vote for increased cancer research funding, and to help "put the nation's fight against cancer back on track." At each meeting—some in the tents, when elected officials

This page and opposite: Politicians from Barack Obama (above)—then a U.S. senator—and Sen. Saxby Chambliss (top right) to Former Speaker of the House Newt Gingrich (top left) and Sen. Dick Durbin (bottom right), and celebrities such as former network newsman Sam Donaldson (bottom left) joined together at Celebration on the Hill in 2006. Opposite bottom right: Sen. Dick Durbin's signature on a proclamation supporting the fight against cancer

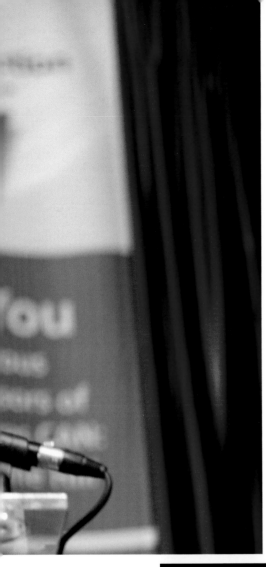

descended from Capitol Hill to meet the advocates on their own turf, some in the marble hallways of the Senate and House office buildings—Celebration ambassadors told their stories, then told their leaders what they wanted. Sometimes there was cheering; sometimes, the strained quiet of people waiting for better answers to their questions.

An Illinois ambassador, standing in the back of his tent and behind his senior senator, Dick Durbin, growled, "If he hasn't signed the promise, he's not going to get out of here until he does. It's free admission, but . . ."

It was an army, all right. And the soldiers could vote.

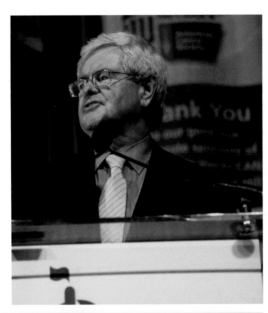

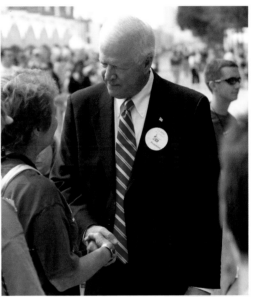

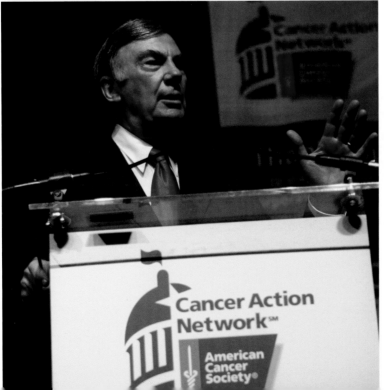

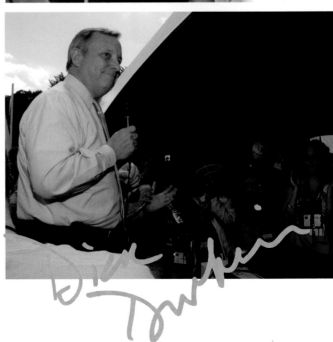

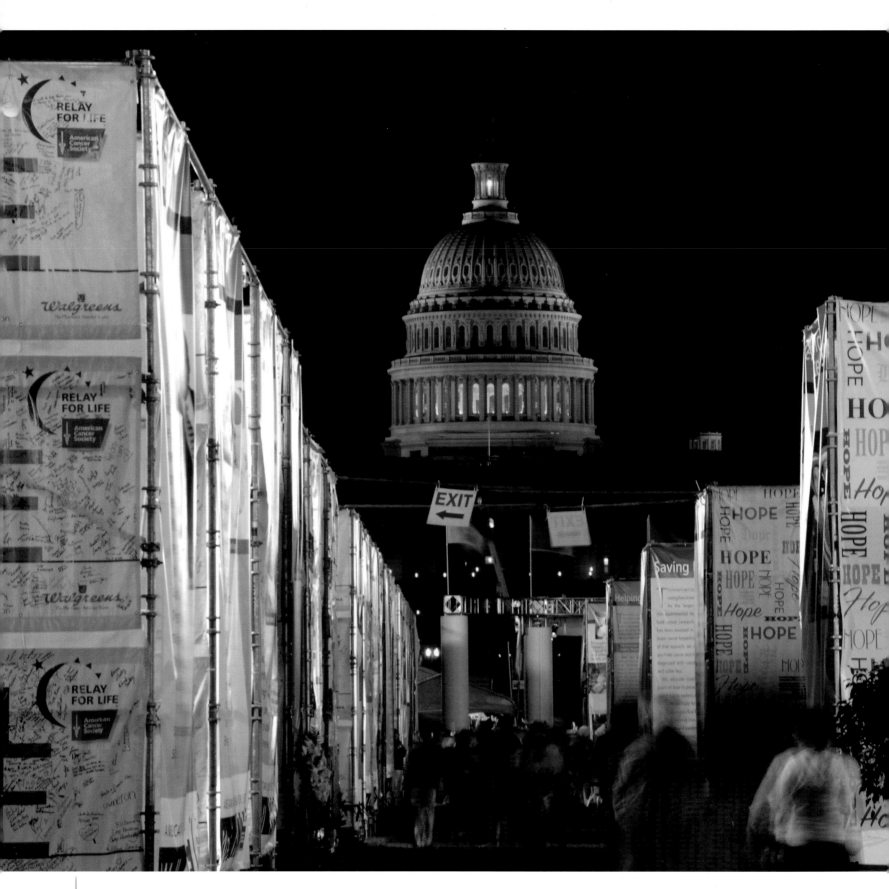

The American Cancer Society

THE WALL OF HOPE

The focal point of the 2006 Celebration on the Hill was the Wall of Hope, which was constructed onsite for the event. Constructing the monument was no small feat, and the final results were nothing short of amazing.

- Construction began thirteen days prior to the Celebration on the Hill event.
- It required thirty-seven thousand pieces of steel scaffolding.
- It required twenty tractor trailers to deliver the necessary components.
- The final monument spanned four city blocks.
- It contained three million signatures and represented four thousand communities, urging Congress to make cancer a priority.

Opposite and this page: Scenes from Celebration on the Hill. The purple pageantry lasted all day and through the night as supporters signed the Wall of Hope, expressing best wishes, recapturing memories, and urging on the fight.

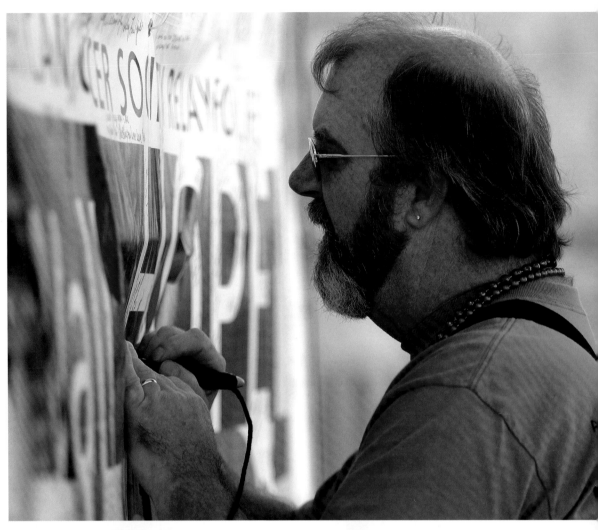

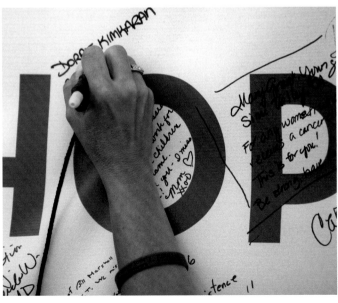

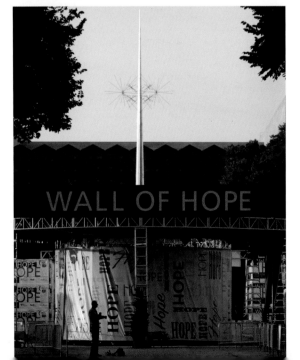

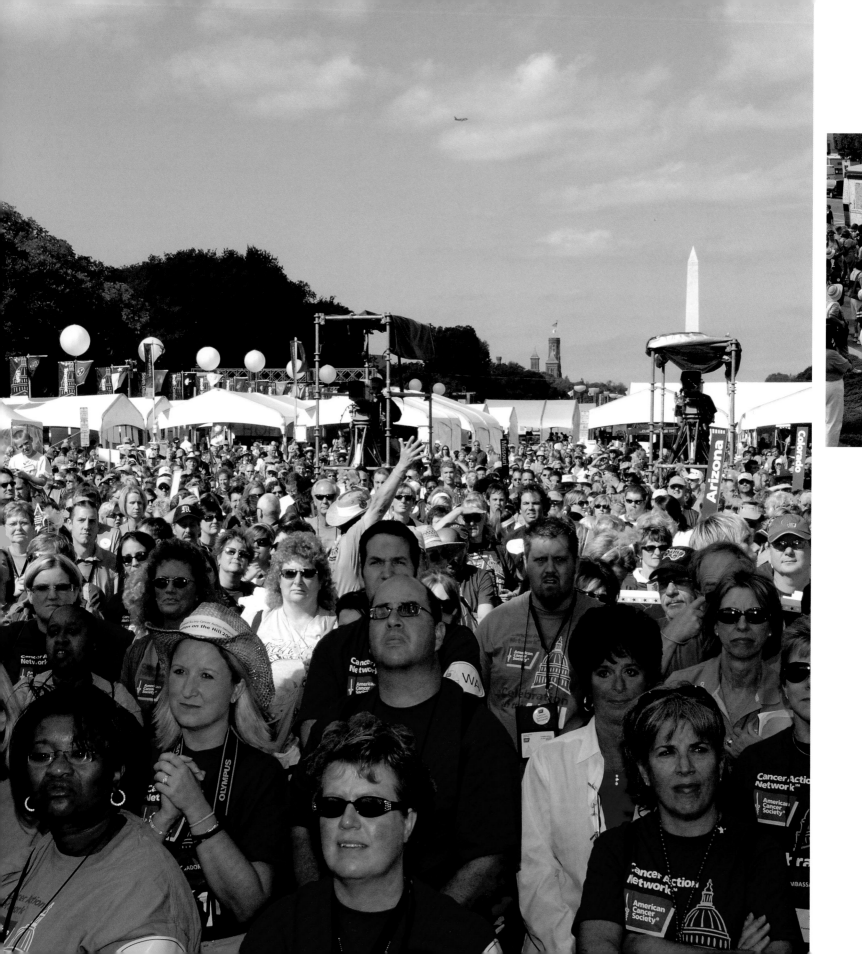

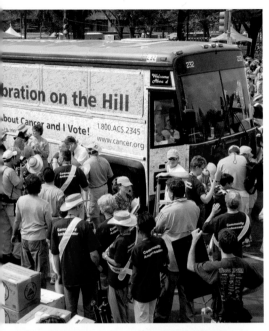

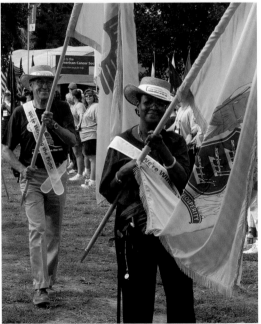

Opposite and above: Some of the more than ten thousand "ambassadors" in the fight against cancer convened for Celebration on the Hill in 2002 and 2006.

"An Untapped Gold Mine"

Celebration on the Hill first came to Capitol Hill in 2002, the first major lobbying effort coordinated by the American Cancer Society. The Society had a vision that this type of event could capture the passion of the fight against cancer that existed across the country. This second event, however, was also a coming-out party for the American Cancer Society Cancer Action Network℠ (ACS CAN), the new advocacy affiliate of the Society.

Using the lessons and strength gathered from the nearly five thousand Relay For Life events held each year, the Society stepped from its traditional path into the hard-tumble world of politics by forming ACS CAN. Because ACS CAN is allowed to take political action, the Society would be affiliated with an organization able to take a stronger nonpartisan role in guiding political decisions that impact cancer. ACS CAN, as the Celebration t-shirts made clear, demanded to be heard at the highest levels.

The move into politics was not a light-hearted one. The Society had already seen how tough politics could be when it became involved in the Proposition 99 fight in California to enact a cigarette tax (see Chapter 5, "The Tobacco Wars"). The Society realized it would be under tremendous scrutiny from the public and the government.

Volunteers like Gary Streit knew that the Society needed to be more involved in influencing political leaders in areas affecting cancer. The Society had tasted political victory in 1988, watching as the California tax increase dramatically pushed down smoking rates. The Society reasoned that an approach like that on a national level might have an equal influence in both anti-tobacco efforts and other areas, but also knew the dangers involved if it entered politics in the wrong way.

The Society had had a small government affairs office in Washington, D.C., for more than a decade. An amalgam of volunteers and staff, the office had grown to about thirty-five people, including Mary Rouvelas, a staff lawyer who helped convince the Society that the formation of a new organization would be crucial in order to protect the organization's interests.

Daniel Smith, former chief of staff for Senator Tom Harkin of Iowa, and current president of ACS CAN, describes his initial impressions of the Society: "When I worked on the Hill, I had done a lot of political campaigns. The Society was like an untapped gold mine from a political organizer's point of view." What Smith saw was Relay For Life, and the tremendous grassroots power Relay gave the Society (see Chapter 7, "Victory Laps"). This was a chance to manage "the mother of all campaigns," with the money and people to do it, unusual for a grassroots organization.

To make the most effective use of its advocacy potential, the Society began creating a new organization entirely. The IRS designation of a 501(c)(4) social welfare organization would allow ACS CAN to engage in more voter education and issue campaigns aimed at influencing candidates and lawmakers to support laws and policies that help people fight cancer. The Society itself is a 501(c)(3) charity, prohibited from engaging in politics.

At the same time, the board expressed concern initially about forming a 501(c)(4). The Society had always prided itself on staying away from politics—although, in truth, it had waged unofficial political battles as far back as 1945 and had used all sorts of political maneuvering to get the National Cancer Act passed in

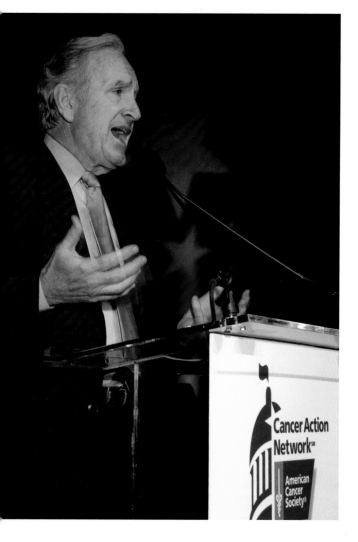

the 1970s. Moving out in the open with those efforts seemed risky; bringing the wrath of politicians onto their heads was nothing the board members thought they wanted to do.

Streit chaired a special commission studying the 501(c)(4) approach and its potential gains and risks. The results were brought back to the board, and the potential gains were clear: the formation of a new entity would help protect the Society and would give it the leverage it needed in Congress to effect change.

Laura J. Hilderley, RN, MS, current chair of ACS CAN and Society national board member, remembers those early discussions. "When the concept of ACS CAN was first presented to the board, we readily acknowledged its value and potential impact on our ability to carry out the Society's mission. But there were many questions to address and issues to resolve before committing to such an enhanced advocacy program. How would our public image be affected? What impact would this have on our volunteers and on our donors? How would it be financed?"

The board voted unanimously to authorize ACS CAN. It was incorporated on September 10, 2001—the day before the attacks on America changed the shape of the nation and the organizations that depended on contributions to do their work. ACS CAN was quiet for a couple of years while the Society figured out how to function in this new landscape. In 2003 and 2004, the organization was dusted off, and the

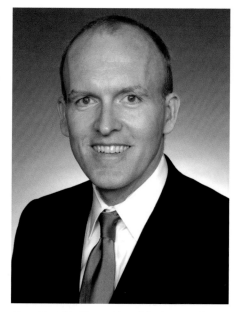

Above: Daniel Smith, president of the American Cancer Society Cancer Action Network. Left: Sen. Tom Harkin (D-IA) speaking at the American Cancer Society Cancer Action Network forum at Celebration on the Hill

American Cancer Society Cancer Action Network began to raise money nationwide. Since then, ACS CAN has supported campaigns across the country to help cities and states go smoke-free and to increase the tobacco tax. ACS CAN used the 2005 New Jersey gubernatorial race as a petri dish to get both major candidates on record on issues important to the fight against cancer. In May 2006, ACS CAN used its grassroots network to generate one hundred seventy-seven thousand e-mails to Congress and to quickly develop grassroots-organized events and press coverage to protest Senate Bill 1955, the Health Insurance Marketplace Modernization and Affordability Act, which would have gutted laws in forty-nine states that require health insurance to cover regular mammograms and other cancer screenings. The campaign produced a very successful "red bra" advertising campaign to support its efforts, which *The New York Times* highlighted in its coverage of the bill's defeat.

Dr. John Seffrin, CEO of the Society

Smith calls the defeat of that bill the "breakthrough moment for ACS CAN. . . . Many of the remarkable achievements in both federal and state tobacco control have come about because of the partnership between Division advocacy efforts and ACS CAN's 'license' to influence legislators." It

was the first time that Congress and other groups in Washington were exposed to the new organization and its impressive grassroots power. "It put us on the map in a whole new way and brought us newfound respect, especially from our opponents in that fight," says Smith.

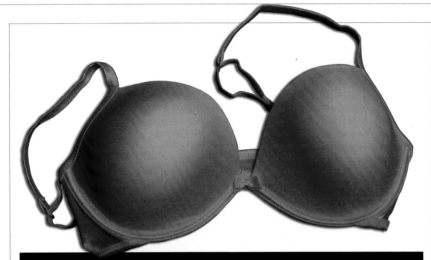

DON'T LET THE SENATE LEAVE WOMEN EXPOSED.

MAMMOGRAMS SAVE LIVES.
HELP US SAVE MAMMOGRAMS.

The U.S. Senate is about to vote on S. 1955, which would gut laws in 49 states that require health insurance to cover regular mammograms. Coverage of other life saving cancer screenings is also at risk.

Tell the Senate to vote NO on S. 1955.
Protect Coverage for Mammograms.

American Cancer Society®

Cancer Action Network℠

1-888-NOW-I-CAN
www.acscan.org

Paid for by American Cancer Society Cancer Action Network℠

Above: The "red bra" campaign was instrumental in a successful effort by ACS CAN to keep mammograms and other cancer screenings covered by health insurance.

A History of Powerful Friends

Powerful friends, and access to them, have been important to the Society in achieving its mission since its formation.

Elmer Bobst, who in the late 1940s became an important and influential supporter of the Society, had known every American president since Teddy Roosevelt. Bobst, the owner of a large pharmaceutical company, was part of a remarkable coalition nicknamed the "benevolent plotters" that had helped get the National Cancer Act of

Elmer Bobst

1971 through Congress and the White House. The passage of the act, the first of its kind in the world, gave attention, funding, and political credibility to the fight against cancer and had been actively supported by the Society.

Pushing the bill through Congress and the White House took discreet political adeptness, calling upon long-forged relationships. Bobst had been a friend of the Nixons for years, so close that the president's two daughters referred to him as "Uncle Elmer." At the same time, Mary Lasker, who had twenty years earlier worked with Bobst to aid in the reorganization of the Society, was a friend and supporter of Democrats, among them Senator Edward M. Kennedy, one of the bill's sponsors. Over the years, she had gathered together a group of people—doctors, politicians, and a renowned Washington society hostess—who spent their

time trying to stimulate federal support of medical research and education.

With Bobst advising the Republican president and Lasker handling the Democrats, the National Cancer Act passed in record time. As the new program unfolded, however, it was clear that the budget was short by at least one hundred million dollars, money the president needed to authorize. Bobst was asked to carry the message to the White House.

When Bobst arrived for the meeting he'd requested with Nixon, he was told the president was running half an hour late. White House administrators knew why he was there, and they knew another one hundred million dollars for cancer research would mean robbing from some other program, perhaps from a political hotspot cooled by the promise of funding for a pet project. They intended to use those thirty minutes to persuade Bobst not to ask for the appropriation.

Bobst realized all this within the first three minutes of the wait. After that, and for the next twenty-seven minutes, he talked, never allowing the aides to direct the conversation toward the one hundred million dollars. After thirty minutes, the door to the president's office opened, and Bobst was ushered in. When he came out, he had a presidential guarantee for the money.

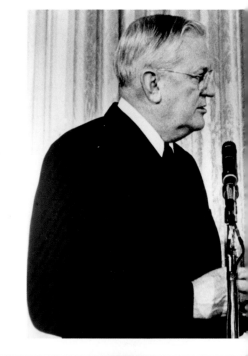

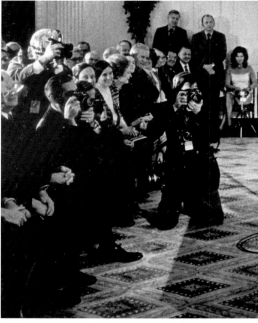

Top: President Richard Nixon meeting with American Cancer Society president, Dr. A. Hamblin Letton, after signing the National Cancer Act legislation. Above: President Nixon signing the National Cancer Act in 1971

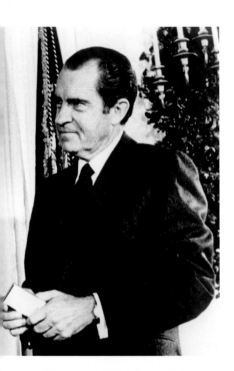

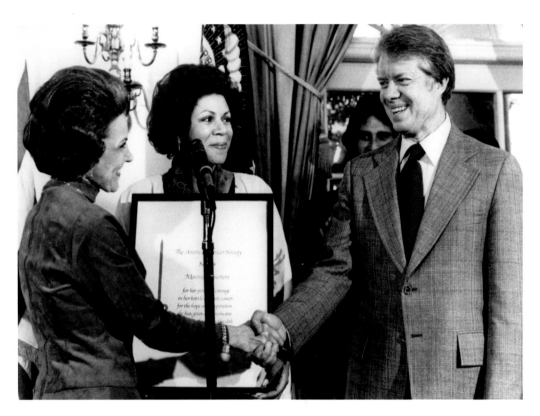

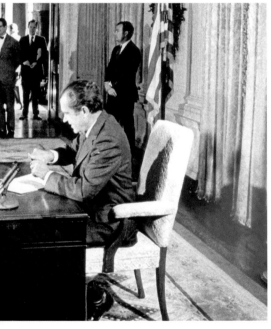

Top right: President Jimmy Carter presents the American Cancer Society Courage Award to Minnie Riperton. Shaking President Carter's hand is Ann Landers, the 1977 National Crusade chairman.

Access to governmental leaders and their support had been an important part of the Society's success. President Warren G. Harding in 1922 endorsed the Society's second National Cancer Week. President Herbert Hoover signed a bill in 1929 making fifty thousand dollars available to the federal Department of Health for fact finding that would aid Congress in drafting and passing legislation for cancer control, in support of the Society's cancer campaign. Franklin D. Roosevelt signed the bill founding the National Cancer Institute in 1937, created with the support of the Society. In 1945, Eleanor Roosevelt was the honorary commander of the Women's Field Army. Dwight D. and Mamie Eisenhower were honorary chairs of the Society's 1962 Crusade. During the last thirty years, the Society has shared the podium with Presidents Jimmy Carter, Ronald Reagan, George H. W. Bush, Bill Clinton, and George W. Bush, each presenting the Society's National Courage Award in the Oval Office to those exhibiting inspiration and hope in their own fight against cancer. First Ladies Betty Ford and Nancy Reagan used their breast cancer diagnoses and treatments to educate the public about cancer and to support Society programs.

Legislative leaders at the federal and state level are wooed, consulted, and counted as friends. Within the space of a few hours on a Tuesday afternoon in September 2006, on the eve of Celebration on the Hill, Society leaders and Celebration ambassadors heard from three potential 2008 presidential candidates—Senator Hillary Clinton, Senator Barack Obama, and Newt Gingrich, former speaker of the House of Representatives. Each stressed the importance of supporting cancer research and lauded the Society for its work.

Whereas working with government at all levels has greatly added to the effectiveness of the Society through the years, the organization has also attracted attention and support from many celebrities—from the Duke and Duchess of Windsor to heartthrob Fabio and professional advice-giver Dear Abby. Along the way, media outlets have been supportive and generous as well: the Society held its first television Crusade kickoff in 1962 with an hourlong program on ABC called *At This Very Moment*. Actor Burt Lancaster hosted the show that featured Eleanor Roosevelt, then Vice President Lyndon B. Johnson, Joanne Woodward, Paul Newman, Harry Belafonte, Danny Thomas, and a half-dozen other entertainers. All donated their time.

A C-Change in Thinking

In many ways, high-level friend gathering is done as an extension of the extraordinary volunteer network that the Society has developed over the years. The Society's very earliest efforts were jump-started by an article in the *Ladies' Home Journal*, which in 1913 had one of the largest circulations in America. That first article led to a long-

standing friendship and relationship between the editors of the magazine and the leaders of the Society. *Reader's Digest*, another influential and trusted magazine (which took no advertising at the time, and, therefore, was considered above political and financial pressures) published several pivotal articles through the years on cancer, thanks in great part to personal friendships between Mary Lasker and the *Digest*'s medical writer. Lasker and Emerson Foote, one of Mary's "little lambs" who helped restructure the Society in the 1940s and went on to influence the government's support of medical research, used a chance lunch meeting in 1944 with the *Digest*'s medical writer to persuade her to do an article testing the waters for an intensive fundraising effort. That fundraising drive, spearheaded by Mary Lasker and her husband, Albert, along with Foote and other new lay members of the board, ultimately raised four million dollars for the Society in a single year—four times more than the Society had ever raised.

❧

Movie stars, politicians, reporters, writers, and influential business leaders are often willing partners in the Society's efforts, although sometimes not without a bit of gentle persuasion. Helene Brown, who was given the Society Medal of Honor for public health in 1997, perfected the art of twisting arms—nicely—in her hometown of Los Angeles.

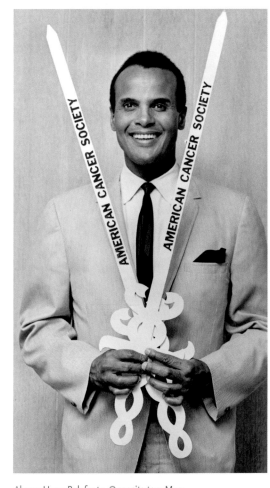

Above: Harry Belafonte. Opposite top: Mary Lasker, who excelled at linking people together in support of the Society. Opposite bottom: President Bill Clinton presents the Society's Courage Award, 1993. With him are Dr. Reginald Ho, national president of the Society, and Stanley Shmishkiss, chairman of the board of directors.

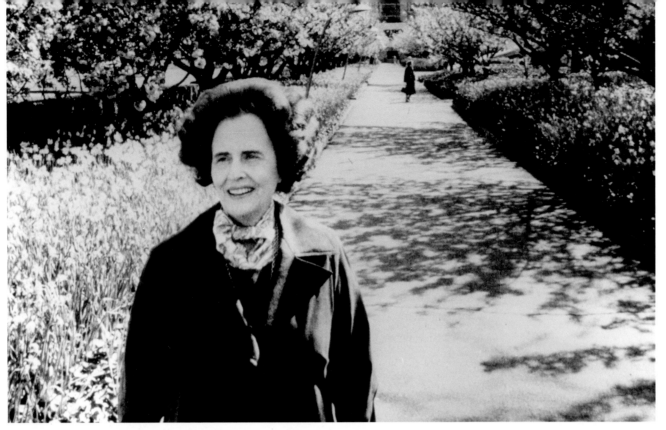

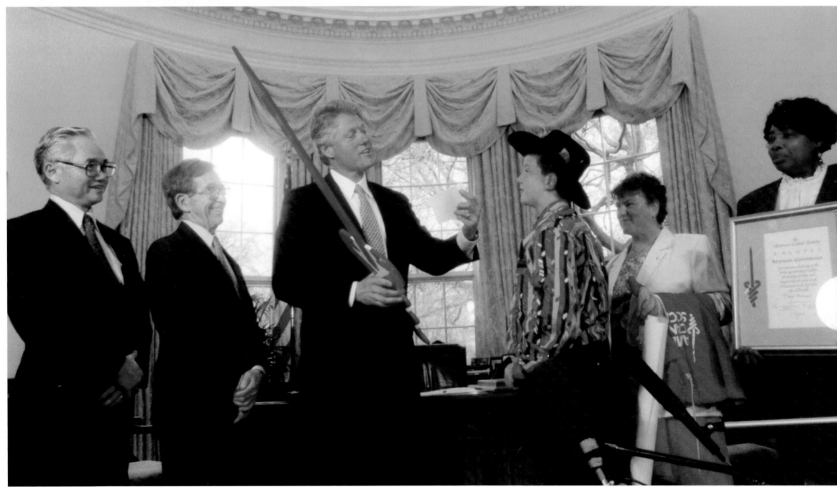

The Stars Come Out for the American Cancer Society

Clockwise this page, beginning right: Reggie Jackson, Engelbert Humperdink, Diahann Carroll, Bob Hope, and Virginia Graham

Clockwise opposite page, beginning top left: The Duke and Duchess of Windsor, Lena Horne, Peter Graves, Joan Crawford, and Rosie Grier

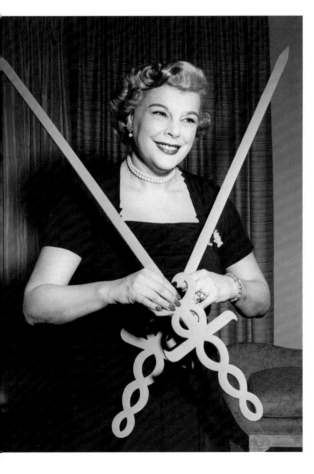

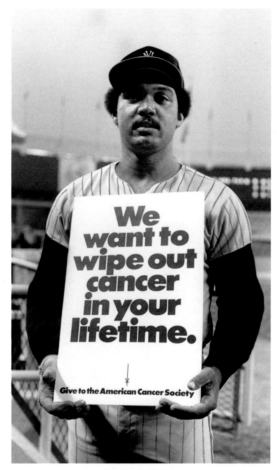

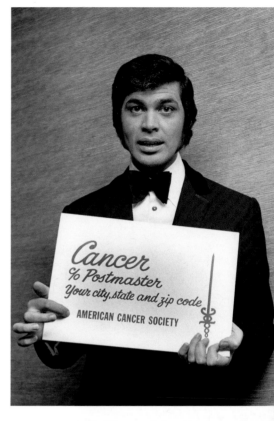

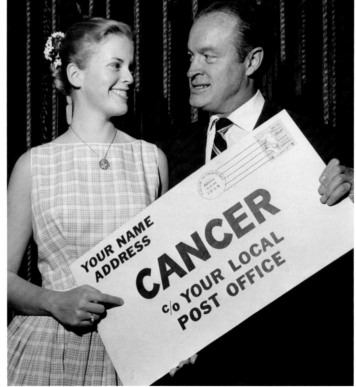

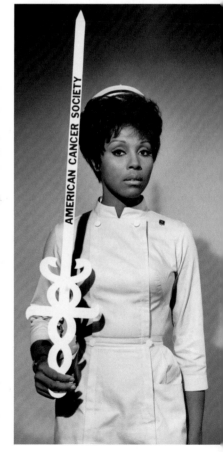

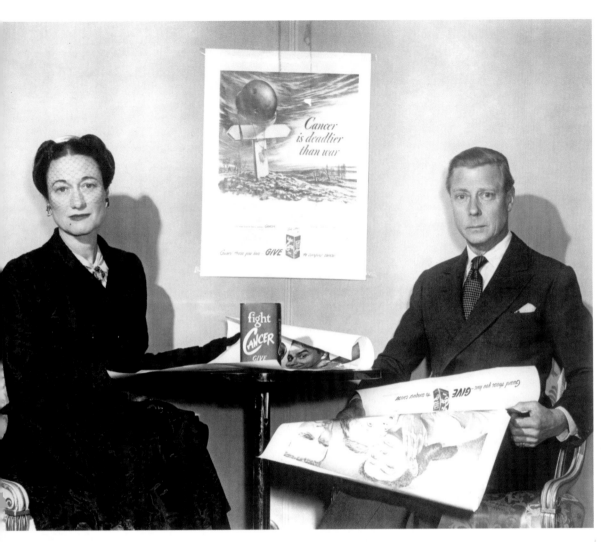

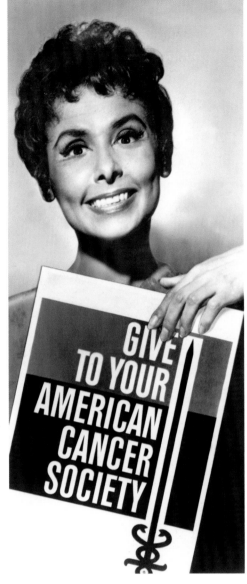

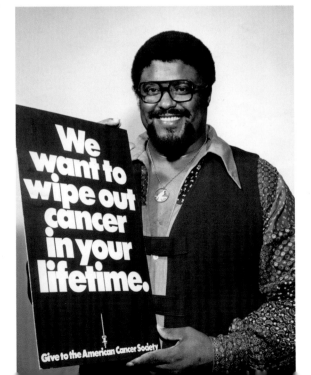

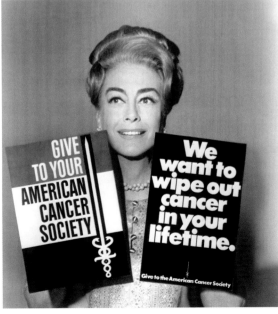

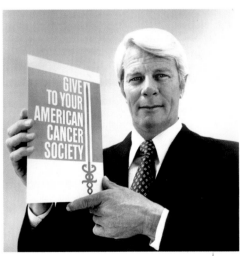

After one lunch with then-Vice President Al Gore, twenty-five top entertainment industry figures, the head of Paramount Pictures, and Jack Valenti (then president of the Motion Picture Association of America), she formed a task force to enlist celebrities to get anti-cancer messages into many venues. "She's a very formidable woman," said Valenti, himself a formidable man who spent almost forty years as the most powerful lobbyist in the entertainment world. "She has a passion for things she cares about, which I find quite laudable."

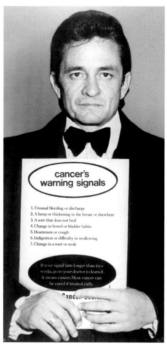

Johnny Cash

And like so many of the Society's volunteers and staff, Brown takes an innovative and refreshing approach to gathering new support. She remembers when Dr. John Seffrin came on as CEO, already talking about twenty years down the road. Deciding that the Society needed expert guidance on such "futuring," Brown donned shorts and tennis shoes and went in search of Alvin Toffler, the renowned author of *Future Shock* and *The Third Wave*. Brown knew he walked the UCLA campus each day, and she was determined to find him, stop him, and ask him whether a health agency could do the same kind of futuring he described in his books. Out of that conversation came

Horizons 2013, which outlines what the Society and the world need to do to control cancer in the future.

Also out of that thinking came the National Dialogue on Cancer, subsequently renamed C-Change, which brought together major organizations, institutions, and groups leading the fight against cancer. C-Change grew out of the growing sense in the Society that there needed to be a cohesive approach to controlling the disease, with three segments of society leading the fight—cancer-specific nonprofits, the private sector (including the pharmaceutical industry), and the government and health care system—brought together for a common good.

"The idea was to get all these people together to start talking, to see if we could find a way to coordinate our efforts on some of the big-picture issues," says Dr. Harmon Eyre, who, with Allan Erickson, a former staff member and longtime consultant, organized the Dialogue. The task was a formidable one with many hurdles to be overcome, including the competition and distrust so rampant in cancer politics.

The Society convened a high-level core group of leaders in April 1998 to develop a report to Congress called *Cancer at a Crossroads*.

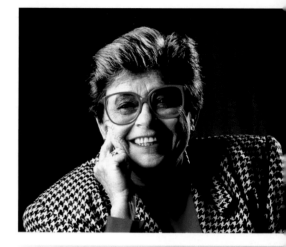

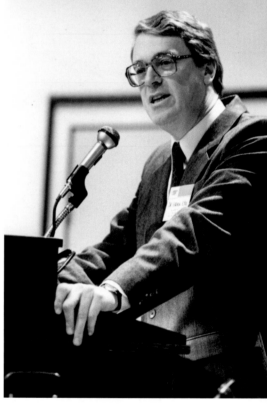

Top: Helene Brown of California has spent more than fifty years as a volunteer and health advocate. Above: Dr. Harmon Eyre, the Society's former chief medical officer, was instrumental in developing the National Dialogue on Cancer. Opposite: *Horizons 2013* outlined what needed to be done to control cancer in the future.

HORIZONS
2013

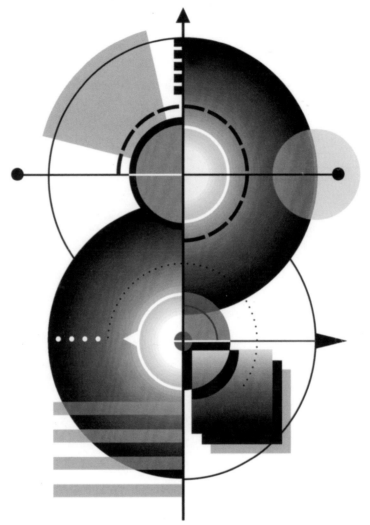

LONGER, BETTER LIFE WITHOUT CANCER

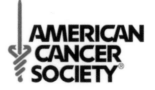

AMERICAN CANCER SOCIETY®

Edited by
Helene G. Brown and John R. Seffrin, Ph.D.
in collaboration with
Institute for Alternative Futures · Clement Bezold, Ph.D.

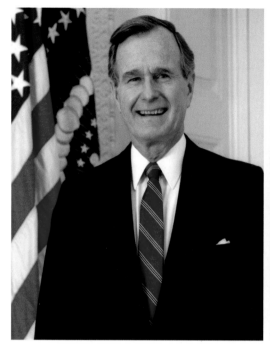
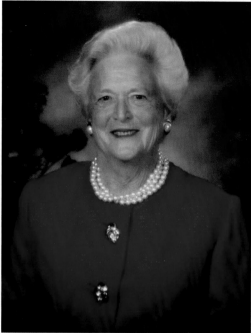
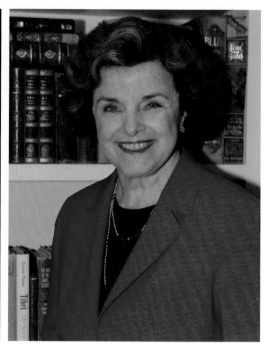

One of the six major concerns delineated in that report was the absence of national coordination of cancer-fighting efforts in the public, private, and voluntary sectors, resulting in service gaps and a costly duplication of effort.

Although the Society initiated the discussion and funded the start-up, the strength of C-Change lies in the credibility of the organizations that joined it and their willingness to become its leaders. Scientists, legislators, media representatives, public health advocates and activists, governmental agency heads, leaders of medical specialty groups, cancer survivors, corporate executives, heads of insurance companies, foundation executives, and opinion leaders of those special population groups that are at greatest cancer risk have all come to the table. Ultimately,

former President George H. W. Bush and his wife, Barbara, became the cochairs of C-Change—which has become an independent IRS-recognized charity—because of their long and genuine commitment to cancer prevention, control, and quality of life for cancer survivors.

Like the Bushes, many of the members of C-Change have long been friends of the Society, deeply interested in health issues and the fight against cancer. Senator Dianne Feinstein—who was the first recipient of the Society's National Distinguished Advocacy Award in 2004, in recognition of her outstanding leadership on cancer issues in the public policy arena—first served as vice chair, and then as chair, of C-Change.

The sense of empowerment that has emerged through C-Change has made its

Above left: Former President George H. W. Bush and his wife, Barbara, became cochairs of C-Change, an IRS-recognized charity. Above: Sen. Dianne Feinstein (D-CA) was the first recipient of the ACS National Distinguished Advocacy Award in 2004 and was chair of C-Change.

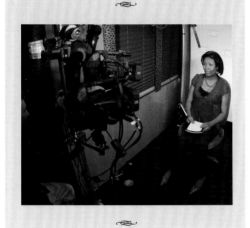

way into business as well as medical circles. A group of CEOs and business leaders from diverse industries founded the CEO Roundtable on Cancer in 2001. United by a pledge to apply the untapped power of business to fight cancer and save lives, the Roundtable was a direct answer to a challenge from former President George H. W. Bush for the CEOs of large companies to do something "bold and venturesome" to defeat cancer. "I called upon CEOs because they are action-oriented people who know how to get things done," says Bush.

The Roundtable has created the CEO Cancer Gold Standard, its first major initiative and an effort that represents a corporate commitment to the health of employees and their families. To attain accreditation, employers must exceed the scope of typical corporate wellness efforts. The rigorous requirements of the Gold Standard call for a company to evaluate its benefits and culture and take extensive, concrete actions in five key areas to promote cancer prevention, early detection, and access to quality care for all of its employees and their dependents in all U.S. facilities.

In April 2006, six organizations received the accreditation necessary to be admitted to the Gold Standard. Among those first being accredited was the American Cancer Society.

C-Change has allowed the Society to widen both its own network and to draw more influential groups into a coordinated effort to fight cancer. "It's a grand experi-

ment in collaboration," Dr. Harmon Eyre says. "It has people talking to each other better than they ever did before."

The Society recognizes that the sort of power it takes to bring people with such contentious competitive spirits together can cut both ways. The Society has been criticized more than once for its connection to corporate interests. In a recent debate, Dr. Michael Thun, vice president for epidemiology and surveillance research, explained the Society's connection to companies engaged in what is often the lucrative field of cancer research. "The American Cancer Society views relationships with corporations as a source of revenue for cancer prevention," said Thun. "That can be construed as an inherent conflict of interest, or it can be construed as a pragmatic way to get funding to support cancer control."

Seffrin and Eyre, in his time with the Society, more than once addressed the issue, pointing out the need to build a better exchange of ideas between the research programs supported by public funds and the pharmaceutical industry—and to help ensure those funds. Bringing those powerful people to the table is as important as having the bipartisan support of presidents for more than eighty years.

The Best and Worst of Reasons

The emotion that cancer generates means powerful friends have been made through the best—and worst—of circumstances.

Paul Rogers, who represented Florida, served for twenty-four years in the U.S. House of Representatives. A leader in Congress when President Nixon signed the National Cancer Act, Rogers served on the Society's board until his death in 2008. Rogers, who earned the nickname "Mr. Health" because of his leadership and advocacy in health issues, was instrumental in helping mend a political rift that might have ended the opportunity to use the National Cancer Act to its fullest capacity. Yet it was his resemblance to another man that solidified his long friendship with the Society.

Dr. A. Hamblin Letton, national president at the time Nixon signed the bill, was mediating between the Society and Paul Rogers's office after the bill was signed. There had been some misunderstandings, and Letton, an engaging Florida "country boy" who had become a well-known oncologist in Atlanta, set up an appointment to try to smooth things over. When he entered Rogers's office, Letton says he thought he was "seeing a younger edition of my father-in-law." As it turned out, Rogers's father and the father of Letton's wife, Roberta, had been in the Florida legislature together and called each other "cousin." Rogers's father and Roberta's grandfather had written the Florida Constitution, and the members of the two families were distant cousins.

Once the pedigrees were established, the two men settled down to working out the problems and found common grounds of agreement. The two couples became close friends, with Rogers referring to Roberta as "Cuz." Rogers became an active volunteer for the Society. Letton himself was so highly regarded by President Nixon that he was offered the job of U.S. surgeon general, an offer he declined.

Sadly, friendships have also emerged from tragedy.

Connie Mack III is a two-term former senator and close supporter of the Society. As a senator, he was influential in achieving crucial budget increases for the National Institutes of Health, a process that took place over five years from 1998 to 2003 and would eventually double the organization's budget.

Mack's brother, Michael, died in 1979 after fighting melanoma for ten years. A decade later, Mack himself discovered a

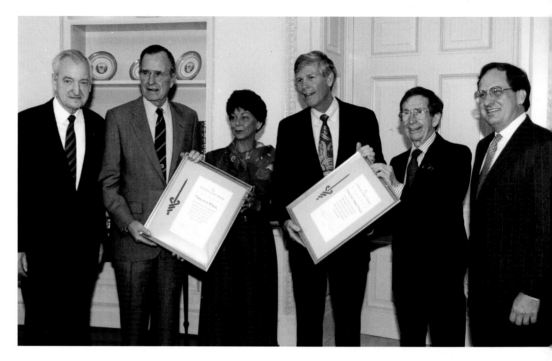

Above: Senator Connie Mack III and his wife, Priscilla Mack, are presented with the American Cancer Society Courage Award by President George H. W. Bush. With them are Dr. Walter Lawrence, national president, Stanley Shmishkiss, chairman of the board, and Don Thomas, chief field officer. Right: Cancer survivors proudly donning their sashes at Celebration on the Hill

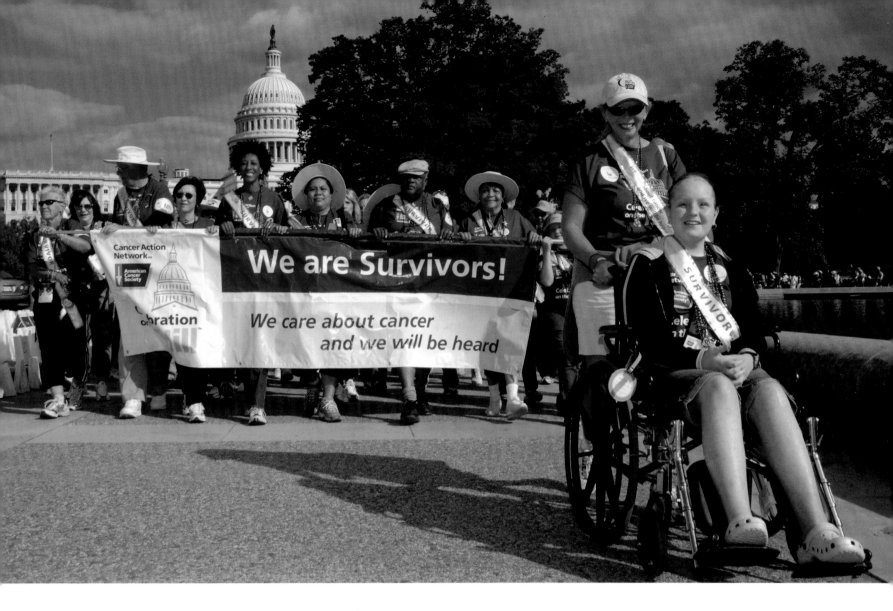

melanoma on his side, which was successfully removed. In 1991, during his first term as a U.S. senator, Mack's wife, Priscilla, found a lump in her breast through self-examination just a few months after a mammogram. She had a modified mastectomy, followed by six months of preventive chemotherapy and five years of tamoxifen, a drug that helps fight breast cancer. His daughter, Debbie, is a cervical cancer survivor. His father, Connie Mack, Jr., died of esophageal cancer in 1996, and his mother survived breast cancer for twenty years, then succumbed to complications of kidney cancer in 1997.

Both Priscilla and her husband became outspoken advocates for the benefits of early detection, and both have been recipients of the American Cancer Society's Courage Award, for those who give hope and inspiration to others.

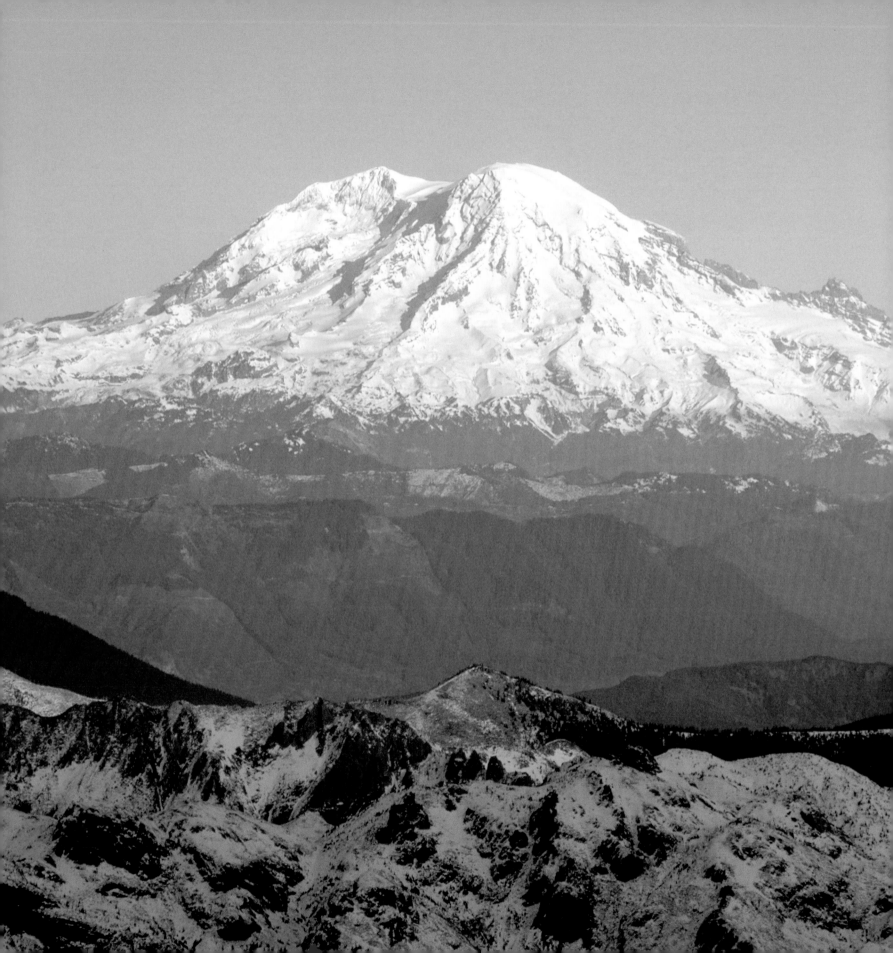

2015 and Beyond:
Moving Toward Victory

CHAPTER TEN

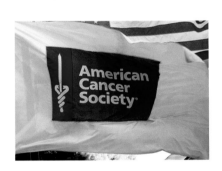

Opposite and above: Mount Rainier, climbed by Darrell Lindgren to mount the American Cancer Society flag, as shown above

Darrell Lindgren climbs mountains. Tall ones, the kind that force humans to confront their own frailties and defeat their own demons. During the last seventeen years, Lindgren has climbed or attempted to climb each of the seven highest peaks in the world. His first climb sixteen years ago was Mount Rainier, a mountain he had studied as a child looking at a book of America's national parks. For a boy growing up in the flatlands of Minnesota, such peaks seemed unimaginable. Although Mount Rainier at 14,410 feet is not among the world's highest, it was high enough to hook Lindgren— a marathoner, musician, and divisional chief financial officer for WellPoint, Inc.—into a whole new sport. And it launched him into a world where the highest peaks of the globe— mountains in places like frigid Antarctica, war-torn Russia, the unsettled jungles of Indonesia—are a challenge to his health, his beliefs, and his dominant will.

He has marked each successful climb with a personal statement: at each summit, he pulls a red, white, and blue flag out of his back-pack and plants it on the mountain.

The flag isn't the American flag. It's the flag of the American Cancer Society.

Why does the Los Angeles resident climb with the twelve-by-eighteen-inch cotton American Cancer Society flag in his pack? For his dad, who died ten years ago of colon cancer. For his friend Patti, who cares so much about

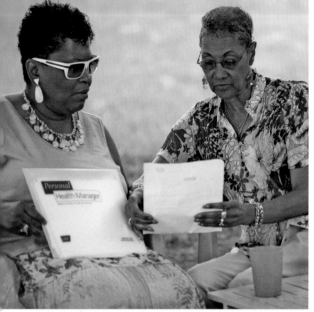

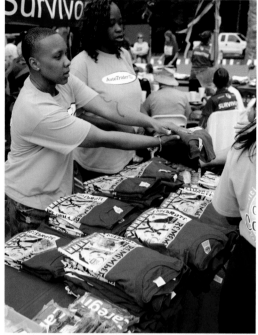

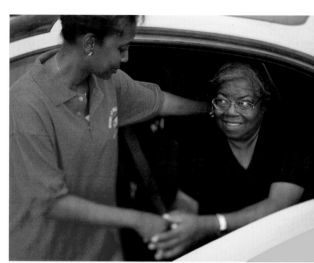

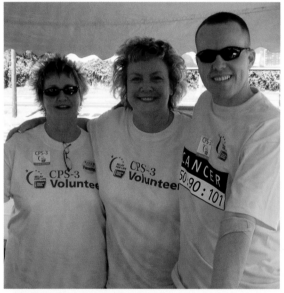

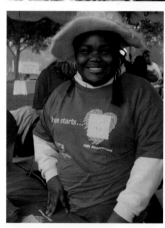

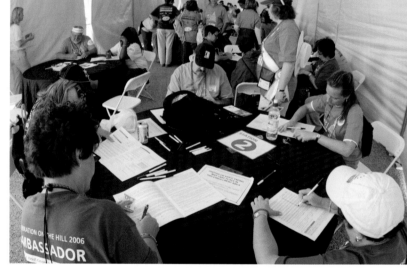

Volunteers have long been the heart of the American Cancer Society. **Top left:** A Reach to Recovery® volunteer talks with a newly diagnosed patient. **Far left center:** Three Cancer Prevention Study-3 (CPS-3) volunteers. **Left:** A volunteer patient navigator talks with a patient and doctor as part of the American Cancer Society Patient Navigator Program. The Society's patient navigators at hospitals and cancer treatment centers serve as personal guides to patients and caregivers as they face the psychosocial, emotional, and financial challenges that cancer can bring. **Upper left center:** Young Making Strides Against Breast Cancer® volunteer. **Above:** Volunteers sign up for CPS-3 at Celebration on the Hill™. **Top right:** A Road to Recovery® volunteer helps a patient out of a car. **Top center:** The color purple was everywhere in Washington, D.C., for Celebration on the Hill, including on these t-shirts being distributed.

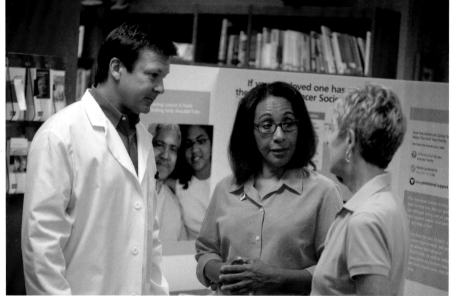

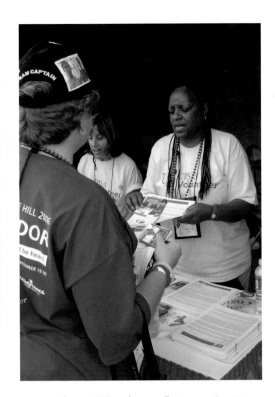

Above: A CPS-3 volunteer talks to a constituent at Celebration on the Hill. Right: Making Strides Against Breast Cancer volunteers distribute apples to participants.

curing cancer. For his own peace of mind. "It's a good organization," he says simply. "I believe in the work it does."

❧

The millions of others who volunteer or work for the American Cancer Society understand what drives Lindgren. It's the same unrelenting passion and vision that push them to find a way to control cancer, the same drive that propels them toward their own summit of sorts: the year 2015.

The American Cancer Society was for decades the sole volunteer-driven agency working for a world without cancer. It was conceived and has survived against all odds. It has tackled the public's reluctance first to openly discuss cancer, then to accept findings that have put some of the responsibility for avoiding cancer on our own shoulders.

The Society has been the most outspoken, most courageous, most stalwart, most successful, most complimented, and most dominant nonprofit organization of its kind anywhere in the world. And, because of that dominance—along with the overwhelming belief that it must overcome barriers, strive tirelessly to succeed, and always offer mercy to others—it has been able to educate and share

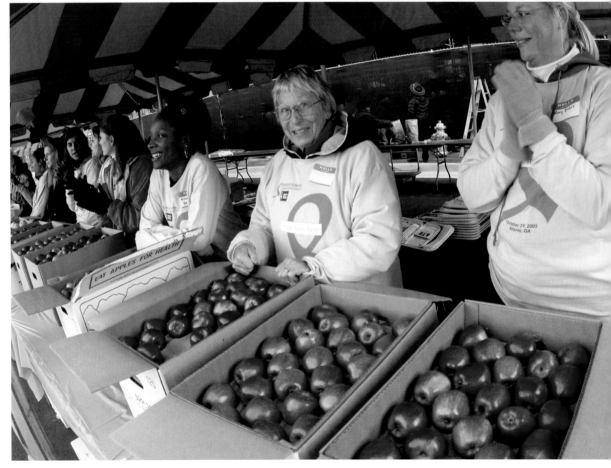

its knowledge around the globe to change the very way cancer is perceived, much less treated.

And Chief Operating Officer Greg Bontrager knows that constantly looking toward the horizon—anticipating and preparing for changes in the world—will ensure the American Cancer Society's ability to remain on the cutting edge of the fight against cancer. "Society as a whole is poised to turn the vision of a cancer-free world into a reality," he says, "and the American Cancer Society is totally committed to that ideal. We will continue to empower people with the knowledge and resources to reduce their risk of cancer, to provide support and advocacy for those patients and families who are already in the midst of the cancer battle, and to fund research that will lead to life-saving scientific discoveries."

As part of that effort to remain on the cutting edge of the fight against cancer, the Society in 2009 launched a historic major brand revitalization effort focused on helping people better connect with the organization and understand all it has to offer to defeat cancer.

"The American Cancer Society brand is iconic in the nonprofit marketplace," says Society National Vice President for Communications Greg Donaldson. "Relevance is key to the health of our brand. This campaign works hard to concentrate and focus the power of this vital organizational asset."

The effort rebranded the Society as The Official Sponsor of Birthdays™, focusing on the many ways the organization saves lives: by

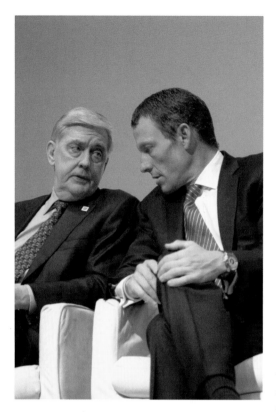

helping people stay well and get well, by finding cures, and by fighting back against cancer.

"The American Cancer Society has a long history of saving lives from cancer—of working to create a world with less of this disease and more birthdays," Donaldson says. "If we can help consumers understand all of the ways we save lives from cancer, we can do even more.

"If we can help more people take steps to prevent cancer and detect it early, if we can increase the number of patients we serve, if we can accelerate our cancer research efforts and engage more advocates in the fight, we believe we can create a world with countless more birthdays."

In July 2007, the Society's national headquarters made another move—this time to a larger building in downtown Atlanta. Later that year, it also became the home of the South Atlantic Division and the Atlanta Regional Office. The building was originally known as the Inforum Technology Center, and the Society became its major tenant, occupying 270,000 square feet on two floors. On October 25, 2007, the building was formally dedicated as the American Cancer Society Center. New neighbors include the CNN Center, Philips Arena, and the Georgia World Congress Center. The downtown location also provides a prime venue for the Society's mission as it works with the city of Atlanta to develop programs that dovetail with the Atlanta Health Initiative.

Left: Dr. John Seffrin and Lance Armstrong. On December 9, 2008, the American Cancer Society, the Lance Armstrong Foundation, and Susan G. Komen for the Cure joined forces with the International Agency for Research on Cancer to release the *World Cancer Report*, which focused on the growing global cancer burden.

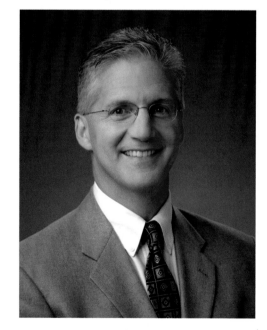

The Society is also looking at how its own organization must be transformed into one that makes collaborations with other organizations an imperative part of ending cancer's oppressive hold over the world's health. Instead of standing alone while raising money, recruiting volunteers, and working to influence laws, the Society has joined forces with organizations such as the American Heart Association and the American Diabetes Association to fight side by side for whole-body health.

As CEO Dr. John Seffrin puts it, "The bottom line is that there's a time for the greater good. We're all interested in improving human health. And I don't think people would be thrilled to think we could eliminate cancer but then diabetes becomes the leading cause of death, when, in fact, some of the same things that can prevent one can prevent the other." Seffrin makes a simple statement—one that would have been unthinkable even a few years ago—that reflects what he thinks can be attained between now and 2015, and then beyond: "Most people don't have to suffer and die of cancer during a normal human lifespan."

In fact, he says, the hopeful side of cancer has never been more hopeful. He knows there will not be a silver bullet that cures cancer. His own life—grandmother

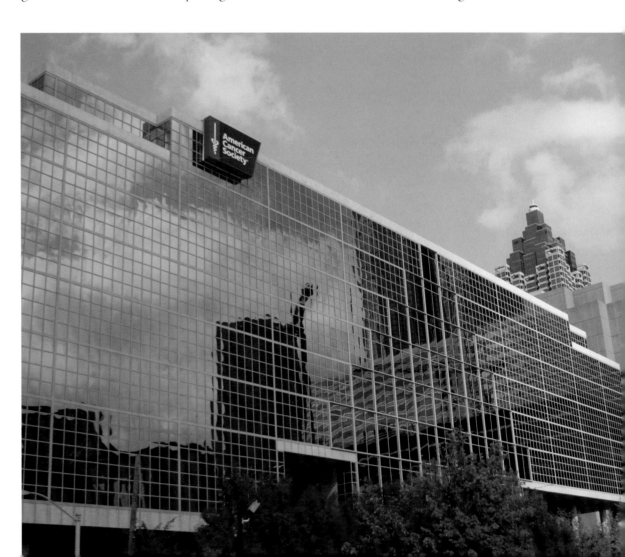

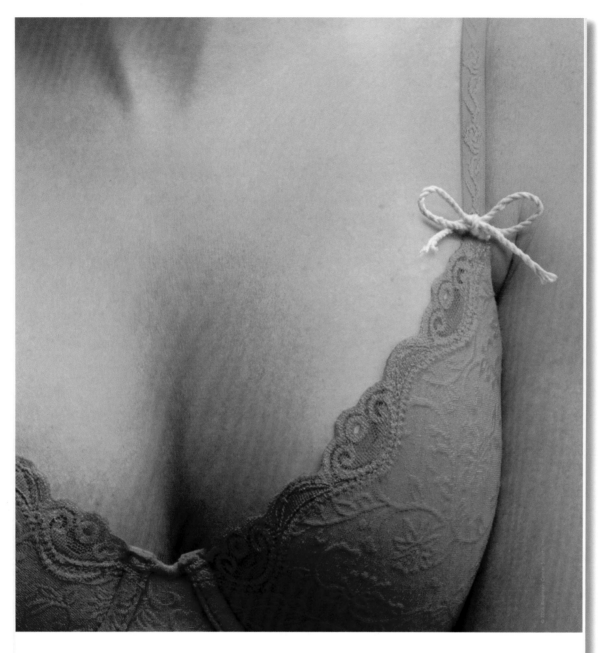

Is it time for *your* annual mammogram?

If getting a mammogram isn't on your priority list, consider this: Research has proven that a regular mammogram is the best way to detect breast cancer when it's most treatable. So in the unlikely chance there is a problem, you can do something about it. If you're 40 or older, talk to your doctor about getting a mammogram. And contact us for a free information kit.

American Cancer Society®

Hope. Progress. Answers.® | 1·800·ACS·2345 | www.cancer.org

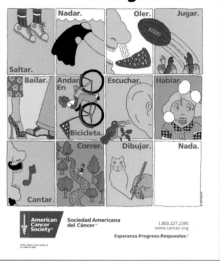

Left and above: Advertisements illustrating the American Cancer Society's emphasis on communicating to the public the importance of the prevention and early detection of cancer

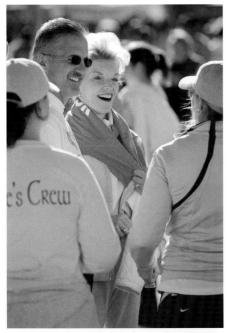

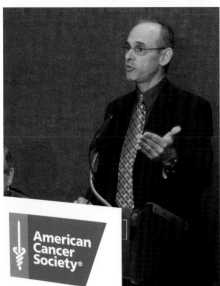

Top: Society Chief Operating Officer Greg Bontrager and Carole Seffrin, wife of Society CEO Dr. John Seffrin and herself a breast cancer survivor, at an Atlanta Making Strides Against Breast Cancer event. Bottom: Dr. Richard Wender started with the Society by publishing a newsletter on prevention. But his dedication to the Society's mission became a lifelong passion: "It added meaning to my life."

dead of cancer, mother dead of cancer, and wife a cancer survivor—is painful evidence of that. But, at the same time, Seffrin has come to believe that it is possible to develop a broad set of strategies to prevent as many as two-thirds of all cancers.

"In the ninety-six years since the American Cancer Society was founded," Seffrin says, "we have taken enormous strides toward unraveling the mystery of cancer. Not only do we know how it develops and becomes epidemic in a population, but we know—indisputably—what it will take to eliminate cancer. Based on our experience and our performance, we have proof of concept that certain measures work.

"Indeed, it's an entirely different world than it was just thirty years ago. When I was in college, acute lymphocytic leukemia in young children was 100 percent fatal. Today, 100 percent of children diagnosed will experience remission, and 80 percent will survive long-term. In the 1970s, only 30 percent of patients survived Hodgkin lymphoma, and no one with advanced disease survived. Period. Today, 80 percent of Hodgkin lymphoma patients will survive. When I was a young man, testicular cancer was 90 percent fatal. Today it's 90 percent curable. Campaigns to build public awareness of the deadly consequence of tobacco use have led to the nation's first declines in lung cancer mortality. So you see that it's not just possible that we can achieve our goals. It's highly likely . . . if we do the right things."

"Doing the right thing" has been at the forefront of Dr. Richard Wender's career. Longtime volunteer and 2006–2007 national president of the American Cancer Society, Dr. Wender first signed on to work for the Society as a young faculty member at Thomas Jefferson University in Philadelphia. He was asked by Steve Weiss, then president of the Philadelphia Division, if he would work on a newsletter for cancer prevention. That was the beginning of a lifelong collaboration with the Society, a relationship that Wender says "added meaning to my life." Today, he acknowledges that prevention and early detection of cancer are very complex. Still the greatest focus of his career, this area of medicine, he says, "involves everything from what physicians should be recommending to their patients, to our culture, our lifestyle and beyond that—to how we run societies, to the political process, to how we pay for health care, to how we help people achieve access to high-quality care, particularly preventive services."

Dr. Seffrin believes the actions that will be necessary to achieve the 2015 goals and continued success beyond include redoubling investment in cancer research. "Thanks to decades of well-funded, peer-reviewed research, defeating cancer is no longer a good bet. It is a sure bet," he says.

Remarkable achievements such as the mapping of the human genome make new cancer cures inevitable, and landmark discoveries such as cancer vaccines, targeted

American Cancer Society
75 Years of History

On June 8, 1989, a time capsule containing items and artifacts from the Society's history was sealed as part of the dedication of the National Home Office in Atlanta. The Capsule will be opened when the disease we know as cancer is entirely cured or controlled. Moved to the Society's new National Home Office in June 2007, the capsule is still adorned with a plaque bearing the inscription, "To Be Opened When Our Task Is Done."

Items Sealed in Time Capsule

Pen used by President Nixon to sign National Cancer Act of 1971
Postage stamp commemorating Dr. Papanicolaou
Package of Camel cigarettes
Women's Field Army hat
75th Anniversary medallion
Vial of 5-FU
T-shirt from Smoke-Free Class of 2000
Tribute to Mary Lasker
American Cancer Society residential kit
152 suggestion letters for time capsule
Exemplar pin
75th Anniversary pin
75th Anniversary promotion kit
CPS I and II questionnaires
Celebration of Life program
Cancer Facts and Figures for Minority Americans
National Women's Conference on Cancer program
National Conference on Meeting the Challenge of Cancer
    Among Black Americans program
American Cancer Society Cookbook
Crusade—The Official History of the American Cancer Society
American Cancer Society Cancer Book
You Can Fight Cancer and Win
Facts and Figures on Smoking 1976–1986
GAS Company kit
GAS Post
"Thank You for Not Smoking" sign
"Smoke-Free Me" button
Gnomes desktop card
Smoke-free Class of 2000 photograph
Report of U.S. Surgeon General on Smoking and Health
Crusade media kit
Crusader kit
How to Examine Your Breasts brochure
Taking Control brochure
*American Cancer Society and the Worldwide Fight Against
    Cancer* brochure
Colorectal cancer brochure
Cancer-related checkup brochure

How to Stay Quit Over the Holidays brochure
Nutrition brochure
Eat Right mass distribution
Breast Cancer Detection project—*CA* Journal
Cancer News
Oncology Nursing Recollection
A Cancer Source Book for Nurses
BSE and the Nurse
Unproven Methods of Cancer Management
R.O.C.K. Camp brochure
1988 House of Delegates and Board of Directors brochure
American Cancer Society—What It Is
Mammogram
Eating Smart booklets
American Cancer Society major policies
Cancer Statistics for 1973, 1971, 1969, and 1968
Cancer Facts and Figures for 1988, 1978, 1968, 1958 and 1952
Photographs of seven U.S. presidents presenting Courage Awards
Annual Report 1947
Annual Report 1987
October 1944 Quarterly Review
1946—Ten Years of Progress of the Field Army of the American
    Cancer Society
Cancer Through the Ages
"Smoking Stinks" button
American Cancer Society contribution container
List of all American Cancer Society presidents, chairs of the board,
    and national executive vice presidents
American Cancer Society logos
Research grant applications
Photograph of American Cancer Society Headquarters on Clifton Road
"I'm a born non-smoker" t-shirt
American Cancer Society strategic plans
Terese Lasser Awards
"We Care" button
Cancer's Seven Warning Signals
Volunteer development button
StreetFight kit
StreetFight button

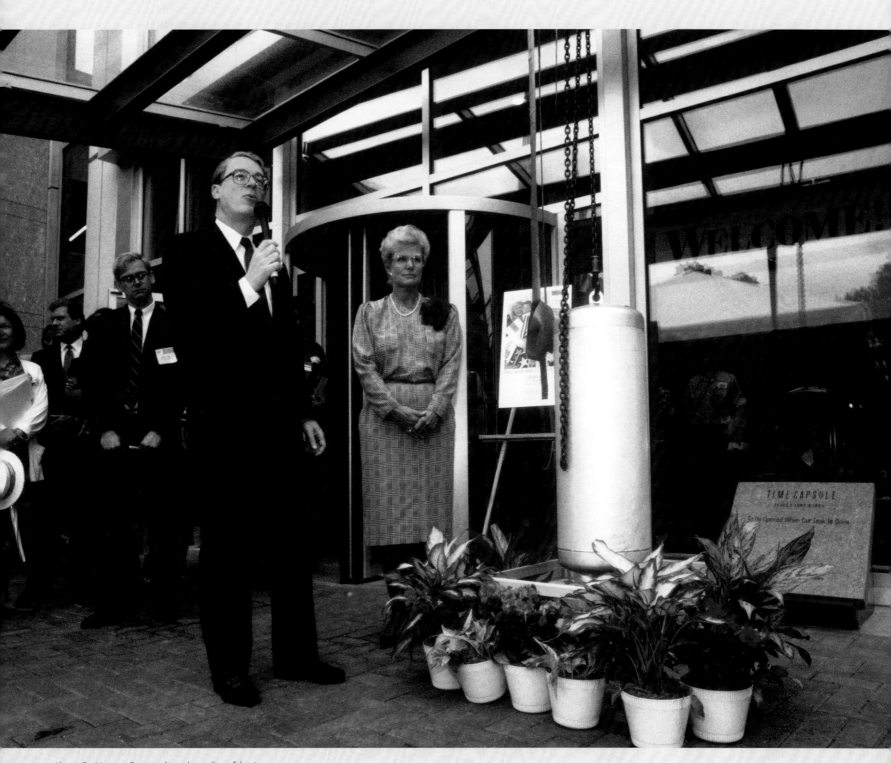

Above: Dr. Harmon Eyre speaks at the sealing of the time capsule. Also pictured is Kathleen Horsch, 1988–1989 chair of the board of directors.

therapies, and chemoprevention are leading to a paradigm shift in how cancer is treated—and translate to thousands of lives being saved every year.

At the same time, Seffrin says, we must make prevention standard practice and public policy nationwide—adopting policies that translate what we know about cancer into what we do about cancer. These policy changes must include bold, aggressive measures such as clean air laws and smoking bans; unfettered FDA regulation of tobacco products and their marketing tactics—especially to children; reimbursement for smokers who use cessation therapies; required health and physical education in all school curricula; increases in tobacco excise taxes, which have been proven to lower smoking rates, especially among youth; and incentives that encourage medical professionals to offer testing to all and that empower citizens of all socioeconomic levels to take advantage of lifesaving screening tests.

Finally, Seffrin stresses the urgent need to ensure that all people have equal access to cutting-edge health care. "With state-of-the-art cancer care, as many as 75 percent of cancer patients could survive long-term," he says. "Tragically, only 60 percent will receive even basic cancer care. If we have the power to virtually guarantee survival, we must work together to make it happen. Preserving and protecting health is a basic human right, not a privilege, but to make it a reality will require funding, attention, and collaboration."

To that end, the Society has already begun to collaborate on what many in the health field feel is going to be the number one issue during the next few decades: universal access to quality health care. The United States is the only developed country in the world that does not provide universal access to health care. Seffrin believes access to care will ultimately be the Society's newest and most dramatic crusade.

"The Society has made progress in delivering on our mission and moving toward our 2015 goals," says Seffrin. "But it has also become increasingly clear that we cannot achieve those goals within the current health care system in this country. Without fundamental change in our health care system that moves toward expanded access to health care, we know we will not be able to achieve our goals."

Dr. Elmer Huerta, 2008 national president of the Society (and the first Hispanic person to serve in that role), has seen what happens when people do not have access to the health care they need. "As doctors, we see direct evidence of how lack of access to care affects patients," he says. "Virtually any doctor who sees patients with cancer in this country knows of people who presented with advanced cancer that should have been found early, but was not. For many of these patients, cost of care and lack of access to care were the main barriers to earlier diagnosis. It is difficult enough for a patient to face a cancer diagnosis without

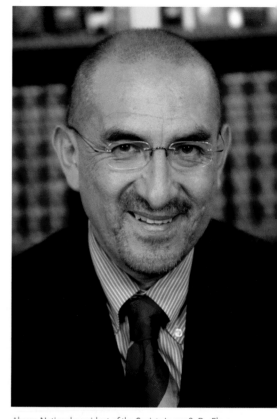

Above: National president of the Society in 2008, Dr. Elmer Huerta has pushed for better access to health care as a means to early detection. Right: One of the Society's advertisements supporting the Access to Care campaign

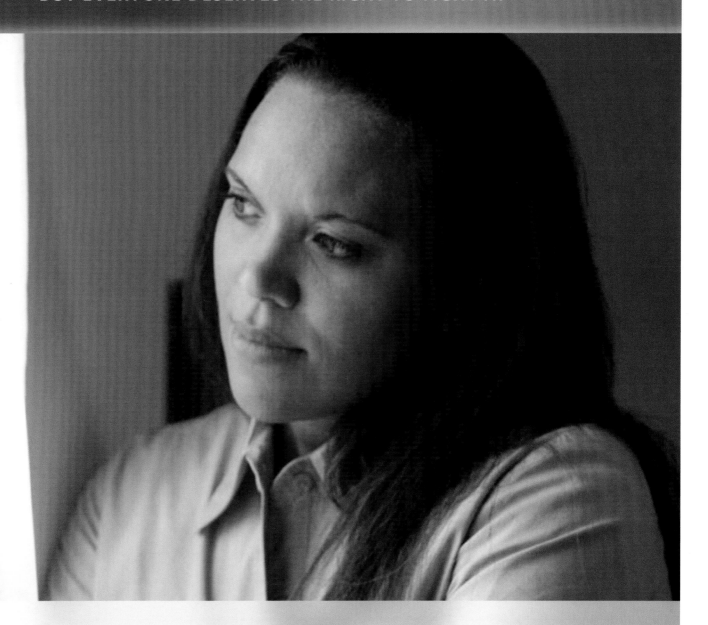

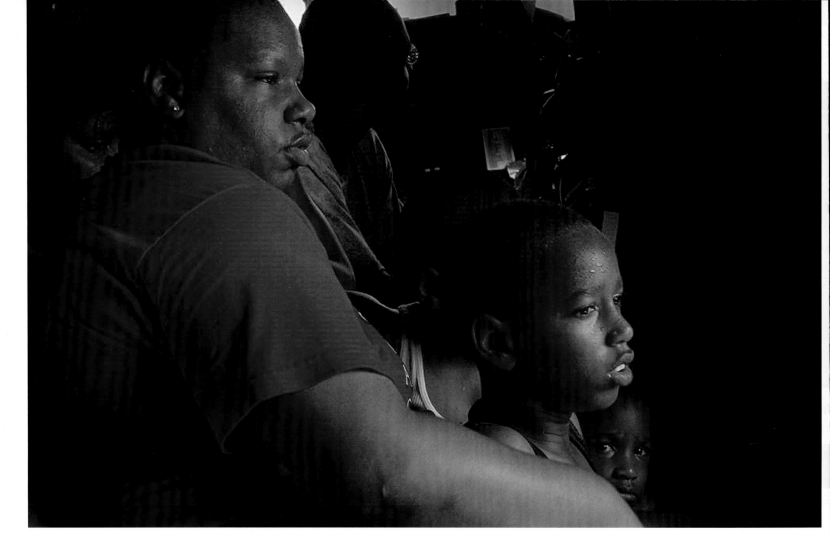

worrying that treatment could put them or their family into bankruptcy or that treatment will be delayed because they cannot find a doctor willing to treat them."

Dr. Otis Brawley, chief medical officer of the American Cancer Society, has focused on health disparities and access to care throughout his professional medical career. A trained medical oncologist and epidemiologist, Dr. Brawley spent years working in inner cities, observing firsthand "what it is like for people who have no access to health care." Most recently, he was recalled to active duty as a military officer with the U.S. Public Health Service in the aftermath of Hurricane Katrina in 2005. For four months, he worked in an infirmary in New Orleans that was adjacent to a "tent city" of more than twenty thousand people. There, he witnessed the overwhelming struggle of people who not only had lost their homes, but had also been deprived of basic health care. In his words, "A substantial number of Americans are being left behind. . . . The United States spends far more per capita on health care than any other nation that keeps such

Above: Hurricane Katrina victims not only lost their homes, but were deprived of access to even basic health care services and thus vital screening services, said Chief Medical Officer Dr. Otis Brawley.

"Cancer is a disease that affects the whole person, the whole family, the whole of our society. Our elected leaders should be addressing the issue by approaching the whole disease."

—Phylecia Wilson, volunteer

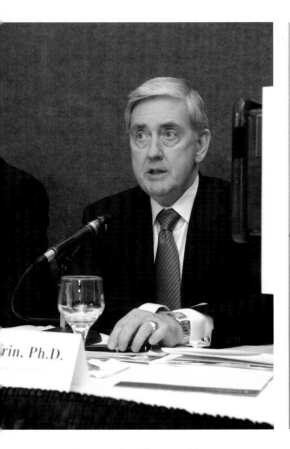

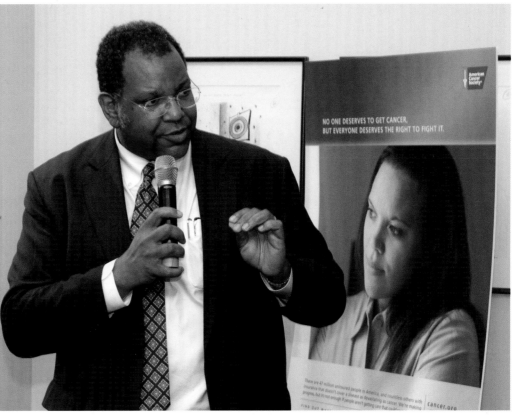

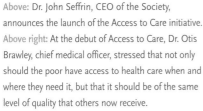

Above: Dr. John Seffrin, CEO of the Society, announces the launch of the Access to Care initiative. Above right: At the debut of Access to Care, Dr. Otis Brawley, chief medical officer, stressed that not only should the poor have access to health care when and where they need it, but that it should be of the same level of quality that others now receive.

records, but lags far behind in life expectancy. Access to care and access to the screening tests that have been proven to save lives are a crucial part of addressing the disparities that exist in our health care system. This is a problem, one that will negatively affect all Americans if it is not solved."

Brawley believes that along with that need to provide access to health care for everyone is the need to ensure quality care for everyone. In other words, the Society's goal is to make sure everybody can get into the health care system when and where they need it and then to make sure that once they have access to the system, they get the same

access to the highest-quality care that only a few now receive.

The Society's goals are indeed achievable when people are empowered to live a healthy lifestyle and to receive proper medical care. For example, cancer mortality is consistently lower among the affluent and well-educated. People aged twenty-five to sixty-four who have sixteen or more years of education are on track toward reaching the 2015 mortality goal. Dr. Seffrin sees this as proof positive that the Society's strategies are sound and potentially lifesaving. "This just shows what can happen if we apply proven interventions so that all people are able to

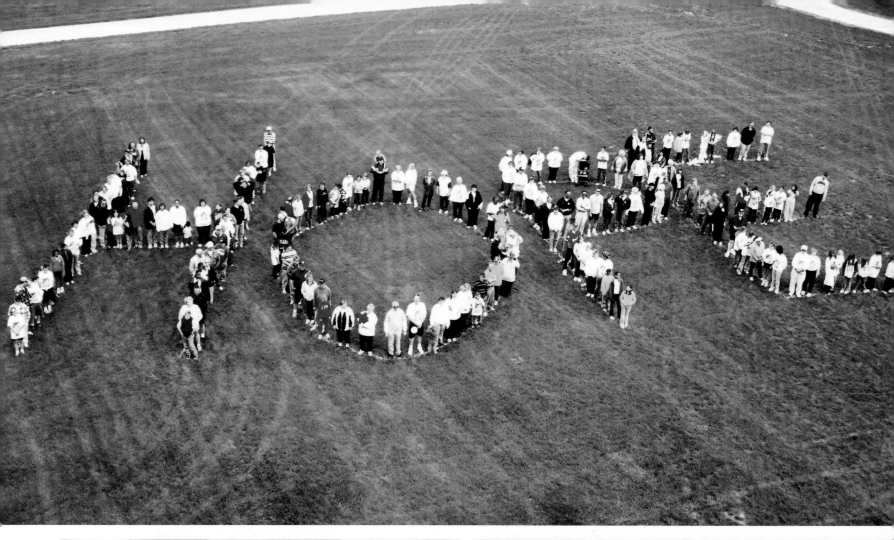

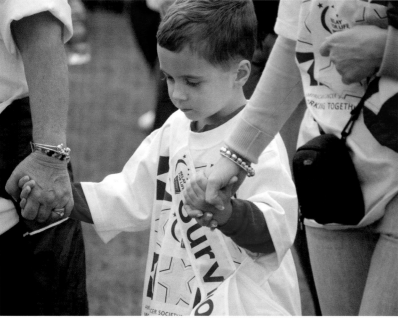

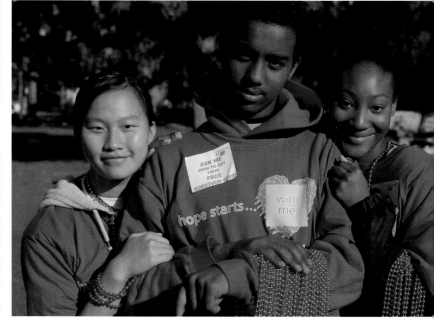

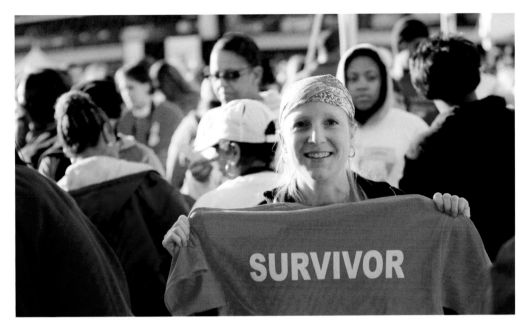

SURVIVOR

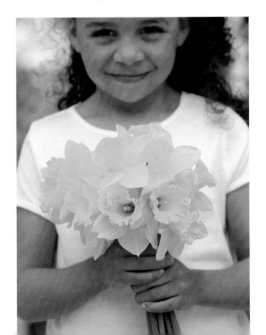

Opposite top: Cancer survivors spell out the critical component of their lives: HOPE. Opposite bottom left: A young cancer survivor at a Relay For Life event. Opposite bottom right: Volunteers at a Making Strides Against Breast Cancer® event. Above: A cancer survivor at Making Strides. Below: A girl holds a daffodil. Daffodil Days® is one of the American Cancer Society's oldest and most beloved fundraising programs. As the first flower of spring, the daffodil represents hope and renewal. To the American Cancer Society, the daffodil symbolizes the hope we all share for a future where cancer no longer threatens those we love.

make the same healthy choices and have the same access to health care as this well-to-do group," he says.

The strategies the Society has developed to control cancer and develop a healthier America are not simple ones. The Society, and subsequently the health care industry, have been likened to a huge ship. Steer it in one direction, and it may slowly find its way through the shoals to a safe harbor. Turn a different way, and the ship runs aground.

"When will the disease be relegated to a very low role? It's the hardest question, because you're trying to project things that are not yet discovered, and trying to project how to change human behavior," admits the Society's former Chief Medical Officer Dr. Harmon Eyre. But the ship is making steady headway toward that safe harbor, and, with each mile that it steams forward, it leaves in

its wake the ultimate reward: lives saved—tens of thousands of them every single year.

Ultimately, the work to lead the American Cancer Society toward and beyond 2015 will not be judged just by politicians, scientists, doctors, and social workers. Instead, it will be judged by people like Nancy O'Barr of Lavonia, Georgia, whose husband, Johnny, stayed for more than a year in the Atlanta American Cancer Society Hope Lodge while undergoing treatment for a rare form of cancer diagnosed when he was fifty. It will be judged by Susan Meyers of West Hartford, Connecticut, who watched her son, Doug, die in his junior year of high school of bone cancer; she began a journey of advocacy that led her onto a stage promising that this "is not going to happen again to others." It will be judged by those who climb mountains with flags in their packs and hope in their hearts.

The efforts will be judged by the people whose lives are spared from cancer and by those who never develop it in the first place. After all, says Seffrin, "Between 1991 and 2005—by doing what we know works—we were able to achieve a 14.4 percent downturn in cancer mortality. That translates to roughly six hundred fifty thousand real people who were able to celebrate more birthdays. And, with our continued hard work and collaboration, those lives are just the beginning.

"We're on the cusp of the greatest public health victory in recorded history," he says. "And may God speed that day."

References

Accomplishments of the American Cancer Society 1945–1999. Atlanta, GA: American Cancer Society; 1999.

American Cancer Society. *Annual Reports*. Atlanta, GA: American Cancer Society; 1952–2008.

American Cancer Society. *Cancer News*. Atlanta, GA: American Cancer Society; 1947–1994.

Articles of Incorporation of the American Society for the Control of Cancer. New York: New York State Department of State, Division of Corporations; 1925.

Baker LH. Breast Cancer Detection Demonstration Project: five-year summary report. *CA Cancer J Clin.* 1982;32(4):194–225.

Ballin SD. Statement on the Protect Our Children From Cigarettes Act of 1989. Washington, DC: Coalition on Smoking OR Health; July 1989.

Bloodgood JC. Treatment delay in breast cancer. *JAMA.* 1924.

Blum A. Counteradvertising. *World Smoking and Health.* 1991;16(3):2.

Bobst EH. Cancer fighting: a rewarding avocation. *Cancer News.* 1954;8(2):10.

Brown HG, Seffrin JR, Bezold C., eds. *Horizons 2013: Longer, Better Life Without Cancer*. Atlanta, GA: American Cancer Society; 1996.

Connolly GN. *Report on the Problem of Smoking*. Washington, DC: Testimony to the Senate Labor and Human Resources Committee; 1990.

Davis AC. The legislative process of the National Cancer Act, 1970-71. Problems and resolutions. *Cancer.* 1996;78(12):2585–2589.

Durant JE. Sword of Hope. Interview. 1954.

Erickson CC. *The Pap Smear Survey Report*. Memphis, TN: American Cancer Society; 1953.

Essential Facts About Cancer. New York: The American Society for the Control of Cancer; 1925.

Evidence of a Causal Relationship Between Tobacco and Lung Cancer. New York: American Cancer Society; 1962.

Graham, EE. *Cancer of the Lung—One Disease*. New York: American Cancer Society; 1953.

Hammond EC, Horn D. Smoking and death rates; report on forty-four months of follow-up of 187,783 men. I. Total mortality. *J Am Med Assoc.* 1958;166(10):1159–1172.

Hammond EC. Remarks on smoking: evidence and ethics. By E. Cuyler Hammond, 1971. *CA Cancer J Clin.* 1988;38(1):59–60.

Hartman WH. *Final Report of the Breast Cancer Detection Demonstration Project*. New York: American Cancer Society; 1984.

Hartman WH. Minimal breast cancer. An update. *Cancer.* 1984;53(3 Suppl):681–684.

Hillhouse A. Strategies to prevent tobacco use by childen. *World Smoking and Health.* 1992;17(3):6–8.

Holleb AI. *Reach to Recovery*. New York: American Cancer Society; 1989.

Holleb AI, Arje SL. The American Cancer Society's professional education conferences. An historical review. *Cancer.* 1971;28(6):1361–1367.

Howe HL, Wingo PA, Thun MJ, Ries LA, Rosenberg HM, Feigal EG, Edwards BK. Annual report to the nation on the status of cancer (1973–1998), featuring cancers with recent increasing trends. *J Natl Cancer Inst.* 2001;93(11):824–842.

Kluger, Richard. *Ashes to Ashes: America's Hundred-Year Cigarette War, the Public Health, and the Unabashed Triumph of Philip Morris*. New York: Knopf; 1997.

Lasser T, Clark WK. *Reach to Recovery.* New York: Simon and Schuster; 1972.

LeMaistre CA. *Smoking and Cancer.* Washington, DC: Testimony before the Senate Health and Environment Committee; 1986.

Manges M. The general practitioner's responsibility in early cancer diagnosis. *Am J Surg.* 1915;29:377–379.

Millay ES. A poet's gift to the American Cancer Society. *Cancer News.* 1953;7(1):9.

Miller LM, Lasker AD. *Cancer News.* 1952;6(4):11, 18.

Miller LM, Monahan J. The cigarette industry changes its mind. *Reader's Digest.* July 1958:35–41.

Morcosson IF. The democracy of disease. *The New Yorker.* May 1940.

New Ideas About Cancer. New York: The American Society for the Control of Cancer; 1927.

Novello AC. Youth: an urgent challenge for tobacco control. *World Smoking and Health.* 1992;17(3):2–5.

Olch PD, Leikind MC. *Landmarks in the History of Cancer Research.* Bethesda, MD: The National Cancer Institute; 1953.

Papanicolaou GN. *The Atlas of Exfoliative Cytology.* Cambridge, MA: Harvard University Press; 1963.

Papanicolaou GN, Traut HF. *The Diagnosis of Uterine Cancer by Vaginal Smear.* New York: The Commonwealth Fund; 1943.

Peck P, Susman E. 40 Years of Fighting Tobacco. *Oncology Times.* 2004;26(5):30, 35–36.

Report of Cancer Prevention Study. New York: American Cancer Society; 1955.

Report on Tobacco. Washington, DC: Federal Trade Commission; 2003.

Rhodes CP. Developing an ACS research program. *Cancer News.* 1947;1(1):3–5, 10–11.

Rigney EH. *A Pictorial History of the American Cancer Society.* New York: American Cancer Society; 1943.

Robbins GF. James Ewing—the Man. The James Ewing Lecture. *Clin Bull.* 1978;8(1):11–14.

Rosenthal E. Study revives debate on need for mammograms before 50. *The New York Times.* May 13, 1992.

Ross WS. *Crusade: A History of the American Cancer Society.* New York: Arbor House; 1987.

Ross WS. *The Climate Is Hope: How They Triumphed Over Cancer.* Inglewood Cliffs: Prentice-Hall; 1965.

Saslow D, Runowicz CD, Solomon D, Moscicki AB, Smith RA, Eyre HJ, Cohen C; American Cancer Society. American Cancer Society guideline for the early detection of cervical neoplasia and cancer. *CA Cancer J Clin.* 2002;52(6):342–362.

Shaughnessy DT. *History of the American Cancer Society* [dissertation]. New York: Columbia University; 1954.

Smoking and Cancer: Some of the Answers. New York: American Cancer Society; 1954.

Sweanor D. Excise taxes in prevention of tobacco use in young people. *World Smoking and Health.* 1992;17(3):9–12.

Sypher SJ, ed. *Frederick Hoffman.* Philadelphia, PA: Xlibris; 2002.

Taylor H. *The American Society for the Control of Cancer.* New York: American Society for the Control of Cancer; 1925.

Terry L. *Smoking and Health.* Washington, DC: U.S. Printing Office, Surgeon General's Office; 1964.

Timothy F. *Report of Reach to Recovery in Europe.* Atlanta, GA: American Cancer Society; 1989.

Trioto VA, Shimkin MB. The American Cancer Society and cancer research origins and organization: 1913–1943. *Cancer Res.* 1969;29(9):1615–1640.

What Every Public Health Agency Should Know About Cancer. New York: American Public Health Association; 1927.

Young R. *Recommendations of the Blue Ribbon Committee on Research.* Atlanta, GA: American Cancer Society; 2002.

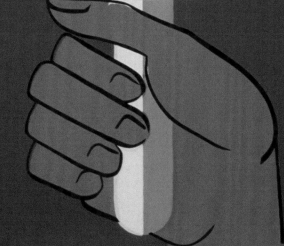

FIGHT CANCER

DELAY IS DANGEROUS

WPA FEDERAL ART PROJECT

CONSULT YOUR DOCTOR OR HEALTH BUREAU

Appendix

AMERICAN CANCER SOCIETY NATIONAL PRESIDENTS

2009	Dr. Elizabeth T. H. Fontham	Louisiana
2008	Dr. Elmer E. Huerta	Maryland
2007	Dr. Richard C. Wender	Pennsylvania
2006	Dr. Carolyn D. Runowicz	Connecticut
2005	Dr. Stephen F. Sener	Illinois
2004	Dr. Ralph B. Vance	Mississippi
2003	Dr. Mary A. Simmonds	Pennsylvania
2002	Dr. Robert C. Young	Pennsylvania
2001	Dr. Dileep G. Bal	California
2000	Dr. Gerald Woolam	Texas
1999	Dr. Charles McDonald	Rhode Island
1998	Dr. David Rosenthal	Massachusetts
1997	Dr. Myles Cunningham	Illinois
1996	Dr. Raymond Lenhard	Maryland
1995	Dr. LaMar McGinnis	Georgia
1994	Dr. Irvin D. Fleming	Tennessee
1993	Dr. Reginal C. S. Ho	Hawaii
1992	Dr. Walter Lawrence	Virginia
1991	Dr. Gerald Dodd	Texas
1990	Dr. Robert J. Schweitzer	California
1989	Dr. Harold P. Freeman	New York
1988	Dr. Harmon Eyre	Utah
1987	Dr. Virgil Loeb, Jr.	Missouri

AMERICAN CANCER SOCIETY NATIONAL PRESIDENTS

1986	Dr. Charles A. LeMaistre	Texas
1985	Dr. Robert J. McKenna	California
1984	Dr. Gerald P. Murphy	New York
1983	Dr. Willis J. Taylor	Washington
1982	Dr. Robert V. P. Hutter	New Jersey
1981	Dr. Edward F. Scanlon	Illinois
1980	Dr. Saul B. Gusberg	New York
1979	Dr. LaSalle D. Leffall, Jr.	Washington, D.C.
1978	Dr. R. Wayne Rundles	North Carolina
1977	Dr. R. Lee Clark	Texas
1976	Dr. Benjamin F. Byrd, Jr.	Tennessee
1975	Dr. George P. Rosemond	Pennsylvania
1974	Dr. Justin Stein	California
1973	Dr. Arthur G. James	Ohio
1972	Dr. A. Hamblin Letton	Georgia
1971	Dr. H. Marvin Pollard	Michigan
1970	Dr. Jonathan E. Rhoads	Pennsylvania
1969	Dr. Sidney Farber	Massachusetts
1968	Dr. Roger A. Harvey	Illinois
1967	Dr. Ashbel C. Williams	Florida
1966	Dr. Leonard W. Larson	North Dakota
1965	Dr. Murray M. Copeland	Texas
1964	Dr. Wendell G. Scott	Missouri
1963	Dr. I. S. Ravdin	Pennsylvania
1962	Dr. Thomas Carlile	Washington
1961	Dr. John W. Cline	California
1960	Dr. Warren H. Cole	Illinois

AMERICAN CANCER SOCIETY NATIONAL PRESIDENTS

1959	Dr. Eugene P. Pendergrass	Pennsylvania
1958	Dr. Lowell T. Coggeshall	Illinois
1957	Dr. David A. Wood	California
1956	Dr. G. V. Brindley	Texas
1955	Dr. Howard C. Taylor, Jr.	New York
1954	Dr. Alfred M. Pompa	Idaho
1953	Dr. Harry M. Nelson	Michigan
1952	Dr. Charles C. Lund	Massachusetts
1951	Dr. Guy Aud	Kentucky
1950	Dr. Alton Ochsner	Louisiana
1949	Dr. C. C. Nesselrods	Kansas
1947–1948	Dr. Edwin P. Lehman	Virginia
1944–1946	Dr. Frank E. Adair	New York
1942–1943	Dr. Herman C. Pitts	Rhode Island
1938–1941	Dr. John J. Morten, Jr.	
1937	Dr. Frederick F. Russel	
1936	Dr. Robert S. Greenough	Connecticut
1934–1935	Dr. Burton T. Simpson	New York
1932–1933	Dr. George M. Bigelow	
1930–1931	Dr. Jonathan M. Wainwright	
1925–1930	Dr. Howard C. Taylor	New York
1923–1924	Dr. Edward Reynolds	Massachusetts
1919–1922	Dr. Charles A. Powers	
1913–1918	Dr. George C. Clark	

American Cancer Society Chairs
National Board of Directors

2008–2009	Van Velsor Wolf	Arizona
2007–2008	Marion Morra, MA, ScD	Connecticut
2006–2007	Anna Johnson-Winegar, PhD	Maryland
2005–2006	Sally West Brooks, RN, MA	California
2004–2005	Thomas G. Burish, PhD	Virginia
2003–2004	Gary J. Streit	Iowa
2002–2003	David M. Zacks	Georgia
2001–2002	H. Fred Mickelson	Oregon
2000–2001	John C. Baity	New York
1999–2000	John R. Kelly, PhD	Mississippi
1998–1999	Francis L. Coolidge	Massachusetts
1997–1998	Jennie R. Cook	California
1995–1997	George Dessart	New York
1994–1995	Larry K. Fuller	Texas
1992–1993	Stanley Shmishkiss	Massachusetts
1990–1991	John R. Seffrin, PhD	Georgia
1988–1989	Kathleen J. Horsch	Wisconsin
1986–1987	Don Elliot Heald	Georgia
1983–1985	G. Robert Gadberry	Missouri
1981–1982	Allan K. Jonas	California
1978–1980	Hon. Joseph H. Young	Maryland
1976–1977	Thomas P. Ulmer	Florida
1974–1975	W. Armin Willig	Kentucky
1972–-1973	Charles R. Ebersol	Connecticut
1968–1971	William B. Lewis	New York
1967	Travis T. Wallace	Texas

AMERICAN CANCER SOCIETY CHAIRS
NATIONAL BOARD OF DIRECTORS

1963–1966	Francis J. Wilco	Wisconsin
1960–1962	Rutherford L. Ellis	Georgia
1953–1959	Governor Walter J. Kohler, Jr.	Wisconsin
1950–1952	General William J. Donavan	New York
1947–1949	Eric A. Johnston	
1946	Ted R. Gamble	
1945	Eric A. Johnston	
1944	Dr. Herman C. Pitts	Rhode Island
1949–1955	Elmber H. Bobst (*Honorary Board Chair*)	

Photo Credits

Foreword

Page viii   Courtesy of the White House

Introduction

Page xiv   Courtesy of the National Library of Medicine/Artist: Charles C. Haight
Page xv   (left) Courtesy of Alabama Department of Archives and History, Montgomery, Alabama
Page xvi   (top) Library of Congress, Prints & Photographs Division, LC-USZ62-61780/Reed & Carnrick
Page xvii   Library of Congress, Prints & Photographs Division, LC-USZ62-106976
Page xviii (right) Courtesy of the National Library of Medicine
Page xix   (top left) Library of Congress, Prints & Photographs Division, LC-F14-00302
Page xix   (bottom left) Courtesy of Harvard Club of New York City

Chapter 1

Page 2   Courtesy of the National Library of Medicine
Page 3   (center) Courtesy of Tokyo University
Page 3   (top right) Courtesy of The Wellcome Trust
Page 3   (bottom right) Courtesy of the National Library of Medicine
Page 4   Courtesy of the National Library of Medicine
Page 5   (left) Cushing/Whitney Medical Library, Yale University
Page 5   (right) Courtesy of Johns Hopkins Medical Institutions/Artist: Thomas C. Corner
Page 6   Courtesy of Johns Hopkins Medical Institutions/Artist: Thomas C. Corner
Page 9   Courtesy of Johns Hopkins Medical Institutions
Page 10   Courtesy of the General Federation of Women's Clubs
Page 11   (right) Courtesy of the National Library of Medicine
Page 12   With permission of the University Archives, Columbia University in the City of New York
Page 13   Photograph by Leonard McCombe/Time-Life Pictures/Getty Images
Page 14   (left) Courtesy of the National Library of Medicine/Photograph by Notman
Page 14   (top right) Courtesy of the Department of Historical Collections, Health Sciences Library, SUNY
           Upstate Medical University
Page 14   (bottom left) Library of Congress, Prints & Photographs Division, LC-D4-33134
Page 15   (top right) Courtesy of National Cancer Institute
Page 15   (bottom left) Library of Congress, Prints & Photographs Division, LC-USZ62-127288/Irving Underhill
Page 15   (bottom right) Library of Congress, Prints & Photographs Division, LC-DIG-npcc-23564
Page 16   Courtesy of The Jackson Laboratory Archives

Chapter 2

Page 21   (bottom left) Courtesy of the General Federation of Women's Clubs
Page 21   (right) Courtesy of The Jackson Laboratory Archives
Page 22   (bottom right) Library of Congress, Prints & Photographs Division, WPA Poster Collection,
           LC-USZC2-1009/Artist: Alex Kallenberg
Page 23   Courtesy of the National Library of Medicine/Photo: WHO
Page 24   (bottom right) Courtesy of the National Library of Medicine
Page 27   (left) Courtesy of the National Library of Medicine
Page 28   (top middle) Library of Congress, Prints & Photographs Division, LC-USZ62-91224/
           Press Illustrating Service
Page 28   (top right) Library of Congress, Prints & Photographs Division, LC-DIG-npcc-04182
Page 28   (bottom right) ©Bettmann/CORBIS

Index

Numbers in *italics* indicate photos and figures.